ACADEMY
POCKET C

Nutrition
Assessment

THIRD EDITION

Pamela Charney, PhD, RD, and

Ainsley Malone, MS, RD, LD, CNSC,
FAND, FASPEN

eat right. Academy of Nutrition and Dietetics

Academy of Nutrition and Dietetics Pocket Guide to Nutrition Assessment, Third Edition
ISBN 978-0-88091-489-5 (print edition)
ISBN 978-0-88091-496-3 (e-book edition)

The views expressed in this publication are those of the authors and do not necessarily reflect policies and/or official positions of the Academy of Nutrition and Dietetics. Mention of product names in this publication does not constitute endorsement by the authors or the Academy of Nutrition and Dietetics. The Academy of Nutrition and Dietetics disclaims responsibility for the application of the information contained herein.

10 9 8 7 6 5 4

For more information on the Academy of Nutrition and Dietetics, visit: www.eatright.org

Contents

Contributors

Pamela Charney, PhD, RD
Program Chair, Healthcare Technology and Management
Bellevue College
Bellevue, WA

Ainsley Malone, MS, RD, LD, CNSC, FAND, FASPEN
Nutrition Support Team, Mt. Carmel West Hospital
Clinical Practice Specialist, American Society for
    Parenteral and Enteral Nutrition
Columbus, OH

Trisha Fuhrman, MS, RDN, LD, FAND
Consultant, Malnutrition Antagonists
Ballwin, MO

Jennifer C. Lefton, MS, RD, LD, CNSC, FAND
Clinical Nutrition Specialist
Medstar Washington Hospital Center
Washington, DC

Mary J. Marian, DCN, RDN, CSO, FAND
Assistant Professor of Practice and Director, Didactic
    Program in Dietetics
University of Arizona, Department of Nutritional
    Sciences
Tuscon, AZ

Susan R. Roberts, MS, RDN, LD, CNSC
Area Director of Clinical Nutrition, Dietetic Internship
    Director, Baylor Scott and White Health, Aramark
    Healthcare
Dallas, TX

Annalynn Skipper, PhD, RD, CNSC, FADA
Health and Science, American Medical Association*
Chicago, IL

Cheryl W. Thompson, PhD, RD, CNSC
MD Informatics, LLC
Carmel Valley, CA

*The information in Chapter 2 is based on the experience and
research of the author and does not necessarily represent the
views of the AMA.

Reviewers

Sarah A. Blackburn, DSc, RD
Clinical Associate Professor; Codirectory IU SHRS
    Dietetic Internship
Indiana University Purdue University at Indianapolis
Indianapolis, IN

Susan L. Brantley, MS, RD, LDN, CNSC
Metabolic Support Nutritionist/Coordinator
University of Tennessee Medical Center—Knoxville
Knoxville, TN

Kay Howarter, MS, RDN
Director, Nutrition Care Process
Academy of Nutrition and Dietetics
Chicago, IL

Mary E. (Beth) Mills, MS, RD, LDN, CNSC
Clinical Nutrition, Nutrition Coordinator RD4
Vanderbilt University Medical Center
Nashville, TN

Acknowledgments

Thank you to the contributors and reviewers of the third edition. We deeply appreciate your commitment to the quality of this revision.

We also gratefully acknowledge the contributions of Gail Cresci, MS, RD, M. Patricia Fuhrman, MS, RD, and Marion F. Winkler, PhD, RD, to the first and second editions, as well as all the insightful feedback from past peer reviewers.

Chapter 1

The Nutrition Care Process

Pamela Charney, PhD, RD

INTRODUCTION

With the introduction of the Nutrition Care Process and Model (NCPM) in 2003, the dietetics profession established a mechanism to communicate about specific interventions unique to dietetics practice. The NCPM serves as a framework to consistently describe the process registered dietitian nutritionists (RDNs) use to think critically and make decisions in all care settings (1–4). As such, it helps RDNs to clearly and systematically articulate the vital services they provide and demonstrate that they are integral members of the health care team.

Patients/clients and other health care providers generally recognize that the RDN provides a unique and highly valued service. However, regulatory agencies and third-party payers are focused on outcomes. When evaluating nutrition care, they ask: "Do RDN services positively impact health outcomes or quality of care in ways that can be documented and measured?" Use of the NCPM helps answer this question through creation of a framework for collecting and analyzing data regarding outcomes of nutrition care.

HEALTH CARE PROCESSES AND QUALITY OF CARE

Avedis Donabedian, MD, is known as the "father of health care quality" (5), and in 1965 he noted that health outcomes are a key component of any assessment of care quality. Donabedian also noted that evaluation of health care quality can be complicated because many outside factors may influence health outcomes. For example, there may be a lengthy time lag between the time of the intervention and significant improvement in the health outcome of interest (6). When health outcomes are not as expected or desired, health care administrators are tasked with determining potential causes. Outcomes can be impacted by something done by the particular health care provider or by *how* care is provided (ie, the care process). For example, a physician might decide that a patient who has a wound infection needs to have a specific antibiotic. The infection might fail to improve because the provider ordered the wrong antibiotic (an issue specific to the provider) or because too much time lapsed between entry of the order and the antibiotic being administered (an issue related to the process of care). Having a standardized care process for a profession, such as the NCPM, helps differentiate between provider-specific causes from process-related issues when evaluating health outcomes.

RDNs are not the only health care providers who utilize a care process to guide critical thinking and decision making in practice. Each of the health care professions has a care process that allows them to delineate the aspects of care that are unique to that profession.

THE NCPM EXPLAINED

In the 2008 visual representation of the NCPM (2), the relationship between the RDN and the patient, client, or group is positioned in a circle at the center of the graphic and surrounded by three rings. The first ring depicts the four steps of the Nutrition Care Process (NCP):

- Nutrition assessment
- Nutrition diagnosis
- Nutrition intervention
- Nutrition evaluation and monitoring

The next ring lists factors intrinsic to the practice of dietetics that affect nutrition care, and the fourth and most external ring identifies concepts that make up the environment in which nutrition care is provided (see Table 1.1) (2). Finally, the graphic shows the screening and referral system and the outcomes management system as outside of the NCP but closely related to it (an arrow points from screening to nutrition assessment; another arrow points from nutrition monitoring and evaluation to the outcomes management system).

Table 1.1   Factors That Impact Nutrition Care

Factors intrinsic to the RDN
- Dietetics knowledge
- Skills and competencies
- Critical thinking
- Collaboration
- Communication
- Evidence-based practice
- Code of ethics

Factors that make up the environment
- Practice settings
- Health care systems
- Economics
- Social systems

Source: Data are from reference 2.

DOCUMENTING CARE USING THE NCPT

Successful implementation of the NCP in clinical practice is supported by use of the Nutrition Care Process Terminology (NCPT; formerly the International Dietetics and Nutrition Terminology [IDNT]). Prior to the development of the NCPT, RDNs would use a variety of words and phrases to describe nutrition problems. In most cases the words and phrases used were accepted and understood by other RDNs and members of the particular health care team. However, providers in other settings may have defined the same terms differently. While convenient at the local level, use of locally developed terminologies made it impossible to correctly aggregate and analyze data from multiple care settings over a wider geographical area.

NCPT is a standardized terminology for the dietetics profession, and use of the NCPT ensures that, regardless of practice setting and geographic location, there is consistent use of words and phrases that have the same meaning (4). For example, data from the nutrition assessment may indicate that intake of food and beverages is not sufficient to meet estimated nutrient requirements. When the RDN uses the NCPT term "inadequate oral intake" to label the problem, it is known that "oral food/beverage intake is less than established reference standards or recommendations based on physiological needs"

NUTRITION ASSESSMENT AND THE NUTRITION CARE PROCESS

As noted above, nutrition assessment is the first step of the NCP. Nutrition screens are used to identify individuals who may have a nutrition diagnosis even though they do not have overt signs or symptoms of a nutrition problem.

If the nutrition screen indicates risk for a nutrition problem, the RDN completes a nutrition assessment to correctly diagnose existing nutrition problems. (See Chapter 2 for more information on nutritional risk screening.)

Nutrition Assessment Components

NCPT terms for nutrition assessment are organized into five domains or categories (4). These are:

- Food/nutrition related history
- Anthropometric measurements
- Biochemical data, medical tests, and procedures
- Nutrition-focused physical findings
- Client history

Assessment techniques for each of these domains are discussed in detail in Chapters 3 through 7 of this pocket guide.

Collecting and Evaluating Data

A great deal of research in medicine and nursing practice demonstrates that novice, proficient, and expert clinicians differ in the type and amount of data needed to accurately diagnose health conditions. At this time there is no reason to think that dietetics practice would differ. Regardless of the amount of information gathered in the nutrition assessment, the goal is to correctly diagnose the patient/client's nutrition problem.

Expert RDNs quickly determine the type and amount of information needed, efficiently gather and evaluate the information, create a "nutrition differential" (list of potential diagnoses), rule out incorrect diagnoses, and correctly diagnose existing nutrition problems. Novice and proficient RDNs are also expected to correctly diagnose nutrition problems but will need additional time and resources. Regardless of the level of practice, RDNs are obligated to refer patients/clients to more experienced practitioners when the situation is outside their area of practice and experience.

What and How Much Data To Collect

Accurate and efficient diagnosis of nutrition problems requires that RDNs determine the types and amounts of nutrition assessment data that should be collected. Although novice and proficient RDNs may need to collect more data than the expert RDN, practitioners at all levels of experience must have an organized approach to data collection.

Nutrition assessment begins with the reason for referral to the RDN and information from the patient history. This information guides selection of the type and amount of data collected. For example, if the patient is not taking any medications, there would be little reason to conduct a detailed assessment of the diet for possible food/medication interactions. On the other hand, if the patient has a recent history of GI surgery, weight loss, and chemotherapy for colorectal cancer, the RDN will focus on data that will help determine the extent and severity of weight loss and the impact of surgery and chemotherapy on nutrient needs, intake and metabolism.

After collecting data, the RDN determines whether data are normal or abnormal. If it is determined that data are abnormal, the clinical significance of the abnormality must be evaluated. The last step before diagnosing nutrition problems is to categorize data. In most cases, an expert RDN completes these final steps quickly. Experience has taught experts how to quickly evaluate nutrition assessment data. Proficient RDNs may complete part of this step efficiently while other parts may require more thought and evaluation. Novice RDNs typically need to take more time to think and consider each alternative while evaluating assessment data.

Regardless of level of practice, the RDN is responsible for determining when enough data has been collected to correctly diagnose existing nutrition problems. Collection of insufficient data may lead to incorrect diagnosis. Collection of extraneous or unnecessary data may lead to incorrect diagnosis and increases costs associated with nutrition care.

NUTRITION DIAGNOSIS

Nutrition diagnosis is the second step of the NCP. RDNs are responsible for correctly diagnosing nutrition problems. A recent search of the Medline database revealed no research focused on thought processes used by RDNs to correctly diagnose nutrition problems. However, there is no reason to believe that RDNs would "think differently" from other health care professionals when diagnosing nutrition problems. Research in medical and nursing education describes several patterns of thinking used to make decisions in patient care. Table 1.2 describes several thought patterns used to make decisions (7–9).

Table 1.2   Examples of Diagnostic Thought Processes

Pattern recognition
- Decision making based on past experience with similar cases
- Most successfully used by clinicians with experience

Exhaustive thinking
- Gathering of as much data as possible followed by search through data for any and all possible diagnoses.
- Typically used by novice clinicians

(continued)

Table 1.2   Examples of Diagnostic Thought Processes
(continued)

Algorithms
- Answers to a series of yes/no questions lead to diagnosis
- Most often used by novice and proficient clinicians

Hypothetico-deductive reasoning
- List of possible diagnoses is developed and altered as information gathering progresses
- Most appropriately used by experienced clinicians

Source: Data are from references 7–9.

Documenting the Diagnosis

Recommendations for documenting and communicating nutrition diagnoses continue to be the least understood part of the NCP. The Academy of Nutrition and Dietetics recommends use of PES (problem, etiology, and signs and symptoms) statements when documenting nutrition diagnoses. This recommendation is based on nursing research that led to creation of the NANDA (North American Nursing Diagnosis Association) nursing terminology (10–12).

When correctly written, the PES statement can clearly and concisely describe what the RDN diagnosed, why the diagnosis was made, and the key finding that triggered the diagnosis (see Table 1.3) (4). Clear, concise PES statements communicate the value of nutrition care to all stakeholders (see Table 1.4).

Table 1.3   What Is a PES Statement?

- A PES statement is written in the form: **Problem** (the nutrition diagnosis) *related to* **Etiology** (the major factor[s] contributing to the nutrition diagnosis) *as evidenced by* **Signs and Symptoms** (the key abnormal finding[s] that determined the nutrition diagnosis).
- Example: Inadequate oral intake related to chemotherapy-related nausea as evidenced by documented intake that is 25% of estimated requirements.

Table 1.4   Tips for Documenting Nutrition Diagnoses

- The PES statement must be clear and concise—it must be easily understood by other members of the health care team.
- Each PES statement must consist of one nutrition diagnosis, one etiology, and one set of signs/symptoms.
- Unless local synonyms have been developed and mapped to the NCPT, terms used should be from the standardized NCPT terms.

Before documenting a nutrition diagnosis, the RDN must be sure that it is correct and contextually appropriate. In many cases, more than one diagnosis could be made. For example, it is not unusual for a patient who has the nutrition diagnosis "overweight/obesity" to also have "Excessive oral intake," "Physical inactivity," and/ or "Food/nutrition-related knowledge deficit." RDNs (or their employer) will need to determine if a PES statement must be written for each diagnosis or if the RDN is able to prioritize and document based on the situation. However, all nutrition diagnoses must be documented—ignoring a nutrition diagnosis implies that the RDN did not correctly diagnose all nutrition problems. Additionally, when nutrition diagnoses are not documented, the implication is that someone else is responsible for nutrition care.

Note: Use of PES statements to document nutrition diagnoses is not required by any regulatory agency. PES statements are one of a number of ways to communicate and document nutrition diagnoses. Each facility should determine how documentation should be accomplished.

Examples

Table 1.5 shows examples of poorly written PES statements followed by revisions to improve clarity. A brief explanation is also included.

Table 1.5   Improving PES Statements

Example 1
- **Original**: Inconsistent carbohydrate intake related to poor diet choices as evidenced by A1C.
- **Improved**: Inconsistent carbohydrate intake related to poor diet choices as evidenced by consumption of 180% more carbohydrate than recommended.
- **Explanation**: The original nutrition diagnosis is not supported by the sign/symptom. A1C is a lab test used to estimate long-term blood glucose control. A1C does not measure carbohydrate intake. Since the diagnosis focused on carbohydrate intake, the sign/symptom must describe some aspect of carbohydrate intake that can be measured in order to determine if the nutrition intervention was effective.

Example 2
- **Original**: Altered GI function related to short bowel syndrome as evidenced by hypoalbuminemia and parenteral nutrition.
- **Improved**: Altered GI function related to short bowel syndrome as evidenced by 7 watery stools per day for previous 5 days.
- **Explanation**: Although there is some thought that the etiology of a nutrition diagnosis should never include a medical diagnosis, in some cases nutrition diagnoses are directly caused by a medical problem. In this example, altered GI function is a logical consequence of short bowel syndrome. Hypoalbuminemia is not a finding that can be directly related to altered GI function, nor will improvement in albumin levels indicate improvement in GI function. Parenteral nutrition is an intervention, not a sign/symptom of a nutrition diagnosis. Changes in stool output can be considered an indicator of bowel function in patients who have short bowel syndrome.

NUTRITION INTERVENTION

Nutrition intervention is the third step in the NCP. After correctly diagnosing nutrition problems, the RDN is responsible for ensuring that the appropriate intervention is carried out.

Ideally the intervention is directly related to either the diagnosis or its etiology. Table 1.6 illustrates this point. See reference 4 for a full discussion of the nutrition intervention step.

Table 1.6   Examples of Correct Nutrition Interventions

Nutrition Diagnosis (Etiology)	Intervention Strategy
Obesity (related to overeating)	• **Correct**: Energy-modified diet: Decreased energy diet • **Incorrect**: Nutrition education—content: Education on low-calorie diet • **Rationale**: The correct intervention is related to the cause of the problem, overeating. Education would treat a knowledge deficit.
Food/nutrition-related knowledge deficit (related to inability to identify lower calorie foods)	• **Correct**: Nutrition education—application: Label reading skills • **Incorrect**: Energy-modified diet: Decreased energy diet • **Rationale**: A knowledge deficit is treated by increasing knowledge.

NUTRITION MONITORING AND EVALUATION

Nutrition monitoring and evaluation is the fourth step of the NCP. In this step, the RDN assesses the patient or client to determine and document whether the intervention has had the desired impact on the diagnosis. Because monitoring and evaluation involves reassessment, the standardized terminology for this step is mostly the same as the NCPT for nutrition assessment. The exception is the Client History domain, which only applies to assessment (because an intervention could not change history). See reference 4 for more information about monitoring and evaluation.

MALNUTRITION DIAGNOSIS AND TREATMENT

The adoption of the NCP and standardized terminology aims to improve nutrition care in all areas of dietetics practice, including the care of patients who are malnourished or at risk of malnutrition. It is generally accepted that malnutrition is associated with increased risk for iatrogenic complications, increased length of hospital stay, and increased health care costs (13). RDNs have always been responsible for correct diagnosis and treatment of malnutrition, although reimbursement for malnutrition was inconsistent. It has only been recently that third-party payers have noted the link between nutrition and outcomes, which is leading to improved reimbursement strategies when malnutrition is correctly diagnosed.

Malnutrition is diagnosed using findings from the patient history and physical examination combined with the RDN's clinical judgment. Recent consensus statements recommend utilization of certain characteristics for accurate diagnosis of malnutrition (14). The NCPT incorporates these characteristics and can be utilized not only to document the nutrition diagnosis "malnutrition," but also to ensure that the role of the RDN in diagnosis and treatment of malnutrition is clearly described. Table 1.7 compares consensus characteristics to the associated NCPT domains (4,14).

Table 1.7   Malnutrition Consensus Characteristics Compared to NCPT Nutrition Assessment Domains

Malnutrition Consensus Characteristic	NCPT Domain
History and clinical diagnosis	Client history
Physical exam/clinical signs	Nutrition-focused physical findings
Anthropometric data	Anthropometric measurements
Laboratory data	Biochemical data, medical tests, and procedures
Food/nutrient intake	Food/nutrition related history
Functional assessment	Nutrition focused physical findings

Source: Data are from references 4 and 14.

REFERENCES

1. Lacey K, Pritchett E. Nutrition care process and model: ADA adopts road map to quality care and outcomes management. *J Am Diet Assoc.* 2003;103(8):1061–1072.

2. Writing Group of the Nutrition Care Process/Standardized Language Committee. Nutrition Care Process and Model part I: The 2008 update. *J Am Diet Assoc.* 2008;1113–1117.

3. Writing Group of the Nutrition Care Process/Standardized Language Committee. Nutrition Care Process part II: Using the international dietetics and nutrition terminology to document the Nutrition Care Process. *J Am Diet Assoc.* 2008;108:1287–1293.

4. Academy of Nutrition and Dietetics. eNCPT Nutrition Terminology Reference Manual. https://ncpt.webauthor.com/pubs /idnt-en. Accessed May 21, 2015.

5. Baker R. Avedis Donabedian: An interview. *Qual Health Care.* 1993;2(1):40–46.

6. Donabedian A. Evaluating quality of medical care. *Millbank Q.* 1966;44:166–206.

7. Croskerry P. Achieving quality in clinical decision making: Cognitive strategies and detection of bias. *Acad Emerg Med.* 2002;9:1184–1204.

8. Coderre S, Mandin H, Harasym PH, Fick GH. Diagnostic reasoning strategies and diagnostic success. *Med Educ.* 2003;37(8):695–703.

9. Coderre S, Wright B, McLaughlin K. To think is good: Querying an initial hypothesis reduces diagnostic error in medical students. *Acad Med.* 2010;85(7):1125–1129.

10. Herdman TH. Nursing diagnosis: Is it time for a new definition? *Int J Nurs Term Class.* 2008;19(1):2–13.

11. Keenan G, Falan S, Heath C, Treder M. Establishing competency in the use of North American Nursing Diagnosis Association, Nursing Outcomes Classification, and Nursing Interventions Classification terminology. *J Nurs Measure.* 2003;11(2):183–198.

12. Gordon M. Nursing diagnosis. *Ann Rev Nurs Res.* 1985;3: 127–146.

13. Agarwal E, Ferguson M, Banks M, Batterham M, Bauer J, Capra S, Isenring E. Malnutrition and poor food intake are associated with prolonged hospital stay, frequent readmissions, and greater in-hospital mortality: Results from the Nutrition Care Day Survey 2010. *Clin Nutr.* 2013;32(5):737–745.

14. White JV, Guenter P, Jensen G, Malone A, Schofield M. Consensus statement of the Academy of Nutrition and Dietetics/American Society for Parenteral and Enteral Nutrition: Characteristics recommended for the identification and documentation of adult malnutrition (undernutrition). *J Acad Nutr Diet.* 2012;112(5):730–738.

Chapter 2

Nutrition Screening

Annalynn Skipper, PhD, RD, CNSC, FADA

INTRODUCTION

Screening programs in health care are a means for clinicians to determine whether a patient or client who has no visible signs of a given health condition may actually have the condition. Screening programs only determine risk (defined as the chance that something bad will happen) for a condition and do not result in a diagnosis.

Accurate and reliable nutrition screening is an efficient means to triage patients according to their need for nutrition assessment and other services of the registered dietitian nutritionist (RDN). Nutrition screening is therefore the entry to the Nutrition Care Process (NCP) and an important component of quality medical care (1,2). Furthermore, nutrition screening is mandated by health care certification and accreditation organizations (see Table 2.1) (3).

Table 2.1   Nutrition Screening Guidelines

- Nutrition screening is referenced in guidelines used by certifying and accrediting organizations. These guidelines are in the State Operations Manuals published by the Centers for Medicare & Medication Services (CMS) for use by their surveyors (3).
- Accreditation bodies such as the Joint Commission, Healthcare Facilities Accreditation Program, and Det Norske Veritas reference the CMS standards when they develop guidelines for institutions and surveyors. It is appropriate to review these guidelines when developing nutrition screening programs.
- In general, nutrition screening must be completed within 24 hours of admission in settings other than long-term care.
- While the specific types of problems screened for may be adapted based on the needs of the institution, certifying and accrediting bodies expect clinicians to rely on authoritative sources to guide practice.

Not all nutrition screens are created equal. Table 2.2 includes some of the characteristics of effective nutrition screens. Table 2.3 defines the terms "false positive" and "false negative" and describes the impact of incorrect screening results. In order to prevent excessive false positive or false negative nutrition screens, nutrition screening programs should be monitored. Prior to initiating screening programs in all care settings, RDNs must determine their "comfort level" with screening results. Is it okay to allow 80% accuracy, or should goals be higher? Once goals for accuracy are set, periodic review of the program will allow adjustment to ensure that patients or clients most in need of nutrition assessment, diagnosis, and intervention receive those services.

Table 2.2   Characteristics of Effective Nutrition Screening Tools

- Simple
- Efficient
- Quick
- Reliable
- Inexpensive
- Low risk to the individual being screened
- Can be completed by any trained health care professional or, in some settings, by the patient
- Has acceptable levels of sensitivity, specificity, and positive and negative predictive values

Table 2.3   Impact of False-Positive and False-Negative Nutrition Screens

Screen Results	Statistical Name	Concern
Positive screen with no nutrition diagnoses present	False positive	Use of RDN time that could be more productively spent with patients requiring RDN services
Negative screen with nutrition diagnoses present	False negative	May not be seen by RDN during typical acute care length of stay

DEFINITION OF NUTRITION SCREENING

The Academy of Nutrition and Dietetics definition of nutrition screening and related considerations is shown in Table 2.4 (4). This definition of nutrition screening replaces an earlier definition of nutrition screening published by the Academy and applies to all populations, regardless of the setting where care is provided or the age of the individuals who receive that care (5,6).

Table 2.4   Academy of Nutrition and Dietetics Nutrition Screening Definition and Key Considerations

Definition

The process of identifying patients, clients, or groups who may have a nutrition diagnosis and benefit from nutrition assessment and intervention by a registered dietitian (RD) or registered dietitian nutritionist (RDN). Patients/clients enter nutrition assessment, the first step of the Nutrition Care Process (NCP), through screening, surveillance systems data, and/or referral, all of which are outside of the NCP.

Key considerations

- Nutrition screening may be conducted in any practice setting as appropriate.
- Nutrition screening tools should be quick, easy to use, valid, and reliable for the patient/population/setting.
- Nutrition screening tools and parameters are established by RDNs, however, the screening process may be carried out by dietetic technicians, registered (DTRs) and others who have been trained in the use of the screening tool.
- Nutrition screening and rescreening should occur within an appropriate time frame for the setting.
- For more information regarding nutrition screening, please visit the Evidence Analysis Library at www.andevidencelibrary.com.

Source: Reprinted with permission from reference 4: Academy of Nutrition and Dietetics Quality Management Committee. Definition of Terms List. www.eatrightpro.org/resources/practice/patient-care/scope-of-practice. Accessed May 6, 2015.

WHERE ARE NUTRITION SCREENINGS CONDUCTED?

Patients and clients are most often screened for nutrition problems in acute and ambulatory care. Nutrition screening is also conducted in ambulatory clinics, in emergency and short-stay units, in long-term care, and in rehabilitation facilities. Because nutrient deficiencies or excesses often exist *before* admission (7) and may not be readily apparent (8), screening for nutritional problems in outpatient settings—including the emergency room, ambulatory clinics—in advance of elective surgical procedures and home care is also important.

WHO PERFORMS THE NUTRITION SCREENING?

Nutrition screening is not typically completed by an RDN, although an RDN is responsible for approving nutrition screening tools, overseeing the training of those who perform screening, and monitoring the screening system. Nutrition screening should be based on data that a nurse or other qualified health care provider, whose knowledge of dietetics is limited, would be able to gather and interpret.

In most acute care settings, nutrition screening is part of the nursing admission process and is required to be completed within the first few hours of admission. Thus it is important that the information needed for screening be available during the initial patient encounter. It is crucial that those who complete the nutrition screening not only do so correctly, but also consistently refer patients appropriately. As health care organizations implement electronic health records (EHRs), RDNs have the opportunity to incorporate the screening and referral process into the EHR.

SELECTING AND IMPLEMENTING SCREENING TOOLS

Clinicians and managers are encouraged to use guidelines from authoritative sources to support practice when appropriate guidelines exist.

Acute Care and Hospital-Based Ambulatory Care

Because validated nutrition screening tools are available, use of tools that have not been validated for screening in acute or hospital-based ambulatory care (eg, SNAQ or DETERMINE Checklist) is not recommended (6,9). An analysis of the evidence supporting various nutrition screening tools is available, and the accurate, reliable, and valid tools it describes are recommended (6). To achieve similar levels of reliability, validity, and accuracy, tools should be used as intended, without modification. If modification of a validated tool is thought to be necessary, then revalidation of the new tool is needed to judge whether or not the modified tool is accurate.

Long-Term Care

In long-term care, the Minimum Data Set (MDS) serves as a nutrition screening form, although validation studies supporting this tool have not been published (10). MDS 3 includes malnutrition in the list of diagnoses that are active on admission. Nutrition information is gathered in section K of the MDS and includes height/weight, weight loss or gain, and need for nutrition support or modified diet. Section K also gathers information on the percentage of energy and fluid needs that the resident has consumed in the seven days prior to admission (11).

Tips for Implementing Nutritional Risk Screening Programs

- Because nutritional status often declines during prolonged hospitalization, protocols should be established to rescreen patients whose initial nutrition screen did not justify referral to an RDN on admission. Each facility must determine the time frame for rescreening, based on average length of stay.
- Appropriate protocols should be in place to ensure consistent and accurate communication of the results of the nutrition screen to the RDN.

- The results of nutrition screening programs should be monitored and evaluated at regular intervals in order to determine whether the screen is accurately identifying those patients who require nutrition assessment and intervention and whether appropriate referrals are being made.

SAMPLE MALNUTRITION SCREENING TOOLS

The Academy's Evidence Analysis Library (EAL) includes a systematic review of nutrition screening tools used in acute care settings (9). Following are brief descriptions of some of the screening tools that were included in the review.

Malnutrition Screening Tool

The Malnutrition Screening Tool (MST) (Figure 2.1) is an example of a rapid screen that can be completed by nurses or other ancillary personnel when a patient is admitted to acute or ambulatory care (12). The MST has been found to accurately predict occurrence of malnutrition when used in acute, ambulatory, and long-term care settings (12–15).

Advantages of MST are as follows:

- It has been tested for reliability and accuracy.
- It is simple for minimally trained persons to use.

When patients are unable to respond to the screening questions, proxy responses from family or caregivers are acceptable. Patients who are unable to answer the screening questions and do not have family/caregivers available should be categorized in the "unsure" category for weight loss and referred to an RDN for further assessment.

Figure 2.1   Malnutrition Screening Tool (MST)

Adapted from reference 12: Ferguson M, Capra S, Bauer J, Banks M. Development of a valid and reliable malnutrition screening tool for adult acute hospital patients. *Nutrition*. 1999;15:458–464. Adapted with permission of Elsevier.

Malnutrition Screening Tool		
Have you lost weight recently without trying?		
	No	0
	Unsure	2
If yes, how much weight in kilograms have you lost?		
	1–5	1
	6–10	2
	11–15	3
	>15	4
	Unsure	2
Have you been eating poorly because of a decreased appetite?		
	No	0
	Yes	1
	Total	

Note: A score of 2 or more = risk of malnutrition.

Malnutrition Universal Screening Tool

The Malnutrition Universal Screening Tool (MUST), published by the Malnutrition Advisory Group of the BAPEN (formerly British Association for Parenteral and Enteral Nutrition), is a five-step nutrition screening tool, which was designed by physicians for use in predicting mortality due to malnutrition (see Table 2.5) (16–18). Its use may be limited if any of the following are true:

- The height and weight of the patient screened cannot be accurately measured (17). (See the downloadable MUST tool [18] for BAPEN's suggestions for alternative measurements and Chapter 4 for more information on measuring height and weight.)
- The patient's weight history is unknown.
- The person conducting the screen lacks sufficient medical knowledge to predict how long a patient will remain NPO based on severity of illness.

Table 2.5   Components of the Malnutrition Universal Screening Tool (MUST)[a]

Step 1: Measure height and weight and determine BMI score
- BMI < 18.5: Score as 2.
- BMI 18.5–20: Score as 1.
- BMI > 20 (> 30 obese): Score as 0.

Step 2: Evaluate recent (past 3–6 mo) unplanned weight loss
- Weight loss > 10%: Score as 2.
- Weight loss 5%–10%: Score as 1.
- Weight loss < 5%: Score as 0.

Step 3: Calculate acute disease effect score
- Patient is acutely ill *and* has had or is likely to have no nutritional intake for > 5 days: Score as 2.

Step 4: Add up scores from steps 1–3 to find overall malnutrition risk
- Score ≥ 2 indicates high risk.
- Score of 1 indicates medium risk.
- Score of 0 indicates low risk.

Step 5: Management guidelines
- For **all** patients, document malnutrition risk category, obesity (if present), and any need for special diets; also, treat underlying conditions and help/advise patients to make appropriate food choices.

(continued)

Table 2.5   Components of the Malnutrition Universal Screening Tool (MUST)[a] (continued)

Step 5: Management guidelines (continued)

- *Treat* **high-risk** patients by referring them to a dietitian or nutrition support team (or implementing other policy), setting goals, improving/increasing nutritional intake, and monitoring/reviewing care plan (weekly in hospital settings, monthly in home or community settings). Note: Treatment is not recommended if nutrition support would cause harm or provide no benefit.
- *Observe* **medium-risk** patients using 3-day dietary intake record. If intake is nutritionally adequate, repeat screening periodically (weekly in hospital, at least monthly in care facilities, every 2–3 mo in community settings). If intake is inadequate or of clinical concern, follow policy for treatment.
- *Provide routine clinical care* to **low-risk patients**.

[a]To download MUST as a PDF file or access the MUST calculator or app, visit: www.bapen.org.uk/screening-for-malnutrition/must/introducing-must.
Source: Data are from reference 18.

Nutrition Risk Score

The Nutrition Risk Score (NRS-2002) in Figure 2.2 is similar to the MUST and is intended to identify patients who will benefit from enteral or parenteral nutrition support (19). It was developed in Europe by physicians and depends on the presence of an accurate medical diagnosis for validity (20).

Since many medical diagnoses are not confirmed until well after admission, this tool may not be appropriate to screen new patients or clients if the admission is for diagnostic purposes. The NRS-2002 also requires more detailed questioning by a health care professional and should therefore not be considered a screening tool, although it is sometimes used for that purpose.

Figure 2.2   Nutrition Risk Score—2002

Adapted from reference 18: Kondrup J, Rasmussen HH, Hamberg O, Stanga Z. Nutritional risk screening (NRS-2002): A new method based on an analysis of controlled clinical trials. *Clin Nutr.* 2003;22:321–336. Adapted with permission of Elsevier.

Nutrition Risk Score—2002	
Impaired nutritional status	
Absent Score 0	Normal nutritional status
Mild Score 1	Weight loss >5% in 3 months *Or* Food intake below 50%–70% of normal requirement in preceding week
Moderate Score 2	Weight loss >5% in 2 months *Or* BMI 18.5–20.5 + impaired general condition *Or* Food intake 25%–50% of normal requirement in preceding week
Severe Score 3	Weight loss >5% in 1 month (>15% in 3 months) *Or* BMI of <18.5 + impaired general condition *Or* Food intake 0%–25% of normal requirement in preceding week

Impaired nutritional status score:_____

Severity of disease (= stress metabolism)	
Absent Score 0	Normal nutritional requirements
Mild Score 1	Hip fracture Chronic patients, in particular with acute complications: Cirrhosis, COPD, chronic hemodialysis, diabetes, oncology

(continued)

Figure 2.2   Nutrition Risk Score—2002 (continued)

Moderate	Major abdominal surgery
Score 2	Stroke
	Moderate to severe pneumonia
	Hematologic malignancy
Severe	Severe head injury
Score 3	Bone marrow transplantation
	Intensive care patients (APACHE 10)

Impaired severity of disease score:_____

TOTAL SCORE:_____

Calculate the total score:

1. Find score (0–3) for impaired nutritional status (only one: choose the variable with highest score) and severity of disease (= stress metabolism, ie, increase in nutritional requirements).
2. Add the two scores (total score).
3. If age ≥70 years: add 1 to the total score to correct for frailty of elderly.
4. If age-corrected total ≥3: start nutritional support.

Mini Nutritional Assessment (MNA)

The Mini Nutritional Assessment (MNA; formerly known as the Mini Nutritional Assessment Short Form [MNA-SF]) is an example of a brief screening tool that was developed and validated for use with elderly patients/clients in community or long-term care settings (21–23). Like the NRS-2002, the MNA was designed by physicians and may not be appropriate for use by nonphysicians in situations where the medical diagnosis is unavailable. Table 2.6 summarizes components of the MNA (21):

Table 2.6 **Components of the Mini Nutritional Assessment (MNA)[a]**

Component	Risk Score[b]
Decline in food intake over the past 3 months[c]	Severe decrease = 0 Moderate decrease = 1 No decrease = 2
Weight loss during the past 3 mo	>3 kg = 0 Unknown weight loss = 1 1–3 kg = 2 No weight loss = 3
Mobility	Bed- or chair-bound = 0 Able to get out of bed/chair but does not go out = 1 Goes out = 2
Psychological stress or acute disease in the past 3 mo	Yes = 0 No = 2
Neuropsychological problems	Severe dementia or depression = 0 Mild dementia = 1 No problems = 2
Body mass index (BMI)[d]	BMI <19 = 0 BMI 19 to <21 = 1 BMI 21 to <23 = 2 BMI ≥23 = 3

[a]To download the MNA form or access the MNA app, visit: www.mna-elderly.com.

[b]A total score of 12 to 14 indicates normal nutritional status; 8 to 11 points indicates risk of malnutrition; and 0 to 7 points indicates that the patient is malnourished.

[c]Decline must be due to loss of appetite, digestive problems, chewing, or swallowing difficulty.

[d]If BMI is not available, use calf circumference (0 = calf circumference less than 31 cm; 3 = calf circumference equal to or greater than 31 cm).

Nutrition Screens Using Laboratory Data (Not Recommended)

Some traditional nutrition screens were based on laboratory data (24). However, laboratory data are not typically available within the time frame specified for nutrition screening (25). Serum proteins such as albumin and pre-albumin are not recommended for nutrition screening because there is no consistent evidence that these markers increase with increased protein intake or decrease with restricted protein intake (9). Thus, nutrition screening or assessment based on serum protein levels is no longer recommended. See Chapter 6 for more information on interpretation of serum protein data.

NEXT STEPS AFTER A POSITIVE NUTRITION SCREEN

If a nutrition screen such as MST, MUST, or MNA-SF indicates that the patient/client may have a nutrition problem, an RDN completes the nutrition assessment, evaluates signs and symptoms, and diagnoses or rules out a nutrition problem (see Table 2.7) (2,19,26). Refer to Chapter 1 for more information on nutrition diagnosis.

Table 2.7   Selected Nutrition Assessment Factors and Related Nutrition Diagnoses Following a Positive Nutrition Screen

Nutrition Assessment Factor	Selected Possible Nutrition Diagnoses
Energy intake compared to estimated energy needs	Inadequate oral intake Inadequate energy intake Malnutrition
Weight change	Unintended weight loss Underweight Malnutrition
Extremities, muscles, and bones	Malnutrition
Body mass index, body compartment estimates	Malnutrition

Source: Data are from references 2, 18, and 25.

SCREENING FOR NUTRITION PROBLEMS
OTHER THAN MALNUTRITION

RDNs must also receive referrals for nutrition problems other than malnutrition, such as the following:

- Vitamin intake—eg, ensuring consistent vitamin K intake for patients treated with vitamin K antagonists
- Obesity—eg, diagnosis and documentation of obesity to support additional reimbursement to compensate for the increased costs of caring for morbidly obese patients
- Knowledge deficits—eg, education focused on modification of sodium and fluid intake, in order to mitigate heart failure symptoms and reduce readmission rates

Adding these criteria to validated screening tools is *not* recommended because changing a validated tool requires that it be revalidated. Furthermore, when using an EHR, it is possible to receive notification of these types of patients outside of the nutritional risk screen.

Pressure Ulcers

There are no studies documenting the prevalence of nutrition diagnoses in patients who have or are at risk for pressure ulcers. However, many believe that these patients are malnourished and in need of medical nutrition therapy. Studies have not been conducted to validate the notion that referring patients to an RDN based on a specific score on a pressure ulcer risk assessment tool is a valid practice. Thus, it is prudent to use valid, reliable, and accurate malnutrition screening tools until published studies demonstrate that presence or risk of pressure ulcers is a better predictor of nutrition problems than the malnutrition screening tools discussed in this chapter.

Anticoagulant Therapy

One of the national patient safety goals of the Joint Commission is to reduce the harm associated with Vitamin K–antagonist therapy in patients who receive these drugs over a long period of time (27). Many programs designed to protect patients receiving these drugs incorporate food and nutrition education. Screening to identify patients taking these drugs may easily be accomplished by computer-generated lists of patients receiving these medications.

Obesity

Screening for obesity can help to identify patients whose obesity increases the cost of their medical care. Facilities providing care for obese patients may receive greater reimbursement for that care if certain documentation requirements are met.

Body mass index (BMI), typically calculated from the admission height and weight, is the basis of the obesity diagnosis (see Chapter 4). The RDN can serve an important role in the screening process for these patients by verifying that the weight used to calculate the BMI is accurate and that the correct BMI is used so that coders have access to that information.

Increased Risk of Readmission for Heart Failure

To help reduce risk of readmission of patients due to heart failure, hospitals may identify patients admitted with a heart failure diagnosis as candidates for nutrition assessment. Screening for high risk for readmission due to heart failure may entail the following:

- Patient history of heart failure
- Presence of edema on admission
- Need for a sodium-restricted diet

REFERENCES

1. Writing Group of the Nutrition Care Process/Standardized Language Committee. Nutrition Care Process Part I: The 2008 Update. *J Am Diet Assoc.* 2008;108:1113–1117.

2. Academy of Nutrition and Dietetics. *eNCPT: Nutrition Care Process Terminology.* 2014. http://ncpt.webauthor.com. Accessed April 15, 2015.

3. Centers for Medicare and Medicaid Services. State Operations Manual. Appendix A: Survey Protocol, Regulations, and Interpretive Guidelines for Hospitals. www.cms.gov/Regulations -and-Guidance/Guidance/Manuals/downloads/som107ap_a _hospitals.pdf. Accessed April 15, 2015.

4. Academy of Nutrition and Dietetics Quality Management Committee. Definition of Terms List. www.eatrightpro.org/resources /practice/patient-care/scope-of-practice. Accessed May 6, 2015.

5. Council on Practice, Quality Management Committee. Identifying patients at risk: ADA's definitions for nutrition screening and nutrition assessment. *J Am Diet Assoc.* 1994;94:838–839.

6. Skipper A, Ferguson M, Thompson K, Castellanos V, Porcari J. Nutrition screening tools: An analysis of the evidence. *JPEN J Parenter Enteral Nutr.* 2012;36:292–299.

7. Coats KG, Morgan SL, Bartolucci AA, Weinsier RL. Hospital-associated malnutrition: A reevaluation 12 years later. *J Am Diet Assoc.* 1993;93:27–33.

8. Singh H, Watt K, Vietch R, Cantor M, Duerksen DR. Malnutrition is prevalent in hospitalized medical patients: Are house staff identifying the malnourished patient? *Nutrition.* 2006;22:350–354.

9. Academy of Nutrition and Dietetics Evidence Analysis Library. Nutrition Screening Evidence Analysis Project. 2009–2010. www.andeal.org/topic.cfm?cat=3584. Accessed April 15, 2015.

10. Centers for Medicare and Medicaid Services. MDS 3.0 RAI Manual (V1.08). www.cms.gov/Medicare/Quality-Initiatives -Patient-Assessment-Instruments/NursingHomeQualityInits /MDS30RAIManual.html. Accessed April 15, 2015.

11. Minimum Data Set (MDS)—Version 3.0 Resident Assessment and Care Screening. www.ncdhhs.gov/dhsr/nhlcs/pdf/train/mds 30resident.pdf. Accessed April 15, 2015.

12. Ferguson M, Capra S, Bauer J, Banks M. Development of a valid and reliable malnutrition screening tool for adult acute hospital patients. *Nutrition.* 1999;15:458–464.

13. Isenring EA, Bauer JD, Banks M, Gaskill D. The Malnutrition Screening Tool is a useful tool for identifying malnutrition risk in residential aged care. *J Hum Nutr Diet.* 2009;22:545–50.

14. Isenring E, Cross G, Daniels L, Kellett E, Koczwara B. Validity of the malnutrition screening tool as an effective predictor of nutritional risk in oncology outpatients receiving chemotherapy. *Support Care Cancer.* 2006;14:1152–624.

15. Cohendy R, Rubenstein LZ, Eledjam JJ: The Mini Nutritional Assessment-Short Form for preoperative nutritional evaluation of elderly patients. *Aging Clin Exp Res.* 2001;13:293–297.

16. Stratton RJ, King CL, Stroud MA, Jackson AA, Elia M. "Malnutrition Universal Screening Tool" predicts mortality and length of hospital stay in acutely ill elderly. *Br J Nutr.* 2006;95:325–330.

17. Malnutrition Advisory Group. BAPEN. Introducing "MUST." Last updated April 27, 2015. www.bapen.org.uk/screening-for-malnutrition/must/introducing-must. Accessed May 5, 2015.

18. Malnutrition Advisory Group. BAPEN. Malnutrition Universal Screening Tool. www.bapen.org.uk/pdfs/must/must-full.pdf. Accessed May 5, 2015.

19. Kondrup J, Rasmussen HH, Hamberg O, Stanga Z. Nutritional risk screening (NRS-2002): A new method based on an analysis of controlled clinical trials. *Clin Nutr.* 2003;22:321–336.

20. Alameida A, Correia M, Camilo M, Ravasco P. Nutritional risk screening in surgery: Valid, feasible, easy! *Clin Nutr.* 2012;31(2):206–211.

21. Nestle Nutrition Institute. Mini Nutritional Assessment. www.mna-elderly.com. Accessed May 5, 2015.

22. Guigoz Y, Vellas B, Garry PJ. Mini Nutritional Assessment. A practical assessment tool for grading the nutritional state of elderly patients. In: Guigoz Y, Vellas B, Garry PJ, eds. *Facts and Research in Gerontology, Supplement 2*. New York, NY: Spraeger; 1994:15–59.

23. Rubenstein LZ, Jarker J, Guigoz Y, Vellas B. Comprehensive geriatric assessment (CGA) and the MNA: An overview of CGA, nutritional assessment, and development of a shortened version of the MNA. In: Vellas B, Garry PJ, Guigoz Y, eds. *Mini Nutritional Assessment (MNA): Research and Practice in the Elderly.* Nestlé Nutrition Workshop Series. Clinical & Performance Programme, vol. 1. Basel, Switzerland: Karger; 1997.

24. Seltzer MH, Bastidas JA, Cooper DM, Engler P, Slocum B, Fletcher HS. Instant nutritional assessment. *JPEN J Parenter Enteral Nutr.* 1979;3:157–159.

25. Kudsk KA, Reddy SK, Sacks GS, Lai HC. Joint Commission for Accreditation of Health Care Organizations guidelines: Too late to intervene for nutritionally at-risk surgical patients. *JPEN J Parenter Enteral Nutr.* 2003;27:288–290.

26. Academy of Nutrition and Dietetics Evidence Analysis Library. Heart Failure Evidence-Based Nutrition Practice Guideline. 2008. www.andeal.org/topic.cfm?cat=2800. Accessed April 15, 2015.

27. Joint Commission. 2015 National Patient Safety Goals: Hospital. www.jointcommission.org/assets/1/6/2015_NPSG_HAP.pdf. Accessed April 15, 2015.

Chapter 3

Food and Nutrition-Related History

Susan R. Roberts, MS, RDN, LD, CNSC

INTRODUCTION

The food and nutrition-related history (FNRH) is one of the five domains of the nutrition assessment (1). The registered dietitian nutritionist (RDN) obtains the information needed for a complete FNRH by interviewing the patient, and/or family/caregivers, having discussions with other members of the health care team, and carefully reviewing the medical record. Table 3.1 describes the components of the FNRH. The Nutrition Care Process Terminology (NCPT) includes terms to describe data collected during the FNRH (1).

Table 3.1   Components of the Food and Nutrition-Related History

Food and nutrient intake
Composition and adequacy of food and nutrient intake, meal and snack patterns, current and previous diets and/or food modifications, and eating environment

Food and nutrient administration
Current and previous diets and/or food modifications, eating environment, and enteral and parenteral nutrition administration

(continued)

Table 3.1   Components of the Food and Nutrition-Related History (continued)

Medication and complementary/alternative medicine use
Prescribed and over-the-counter medications, including herbal preparations and complementary/alternative medicine products used (see Chapter 7)

Knowledge/beliefs/attitudes
Understanding of nutrition-related concepts and conviction of the truth and feelings/emotions toward some nutrition-related statement or phenomenon, along with readiness to change nutrition-related behaviors

Behavior
Patient/client activities and actions that influence achievement of nutrition-related goals

Factors affecting access to food and food/nutrition-related supplies
Factors that affect intake and availability of a sufficient quantity of safe, healthful food and water, as well as food/nutrition-related supplies

Physical activity and function
Physical activity, cognitive and physical ability to engage in specific tasks, eg, breastfeeding and self-feeding

Nutrition-related patient/client-centered measures
Patient/client's perception of his or her nutrition intervention and its impact on life

Source: Data are from reference 1.

USING INFORMATION TO DIAGNOSE NUTRITION PROBLEMS

RDNs should compare data collected during the FNRH to standard or accepted norms (1). For example, if the data collected seem to indicate that the patient may be consuming insufficient amounts of fiber or fluid, the patient's usual fiber and fluid intake should be compared to recommended intake of these nutrients. Data that do not meet the standard or accepted norm must be further evaluated in order to correctly diagnose nutrition problems.

USING INFORMATION TO MONITOR AND EVALUATE RESPONSE TO NUTRITION INTERVENTIONS

The patient's FNRH assists in diagnosing nutrition problems but is also used to monitor and evaluate response to nutrition interventions. Data from the FNRH can help assess whether the patient understands, tolerates, and/or complies with nutrition interventions and/or recommendations (2). Furthermore, FNRH may provide insight into why the patient's nutritional status is not improving despite nutrition interventions. Therefore, it is important to perform ongoing FNRH throughout the individual's continuum of care.

GENERAL GUIDELINES FOR CONDUCTING A FOOD AND NUTRITION-RELATED HISTORY

Each patient is unique, and the RDN should plan the interview to obtain relevant and useful data related to the patient. Obtaining all of the information contained in Table 3.1 from every patient is not a realistic goal. The interview should be tailored to the patient, setting, and the RDN's past experience in similar situations.

Prior to the interview, the medical record should be reviewed to determine factors such as age, gender, medical problems, and medications. Gathering this information can help focus the interview to important areas. As RDNs gain more experience with specific patient populations and medical diagnoses, their awareness of findings that are most often associated with nutrition diagnoses becomes heightened and their skills in conducting a focused FNRH improve.

The interview is more successful if the patient is made to feel comfortable. Consider the following:

- Greet the patient, introduce yourself, and explain the reason for the interview.
- If possible, use a private room to obtain the FNRH.
- If others, such as friends or family members, are present, ask the patient if he or she would like to have the discussion alone or with others present.
- Employ active listening, display empathy, reassure, validate, and empower the patient.
- Use a patient-centered philosophy which includes showing genuine interest in the patient, not just their problems.

COMPONENTS OF THE FOOD AND NUTRITION-RELATED HISTORY

There are eight classes in the FNRH domain (see Table 3.1) (1). Some classes are pertinent to all patients while others will only be applicable in certain settings, such as an outpatient clinic where multiple follow-up visits are possible. For example, it is unlikely that "knowledge/belief/attitude" is relevant for a critically ill trauma patient or for elderly patients with severe dementia in a long-term care facility.

Food and Nutrient Intake

Assessment in the Food and Nutrient Intake domain examines composition and adequacy of food and nutrient intake, in addition to meal and snack patterns. Depending on the patient or care setting, the following might be considered in estimation of food and nutrient intake (1):

- Energy intake
- Food and beverage intake

- Breastmilk/infant formula intake
- Enteral and parenteral intake
- Bioactive substance intake
- Macronutrient intake
- Micronutrient intake

Intake Data Collection Methods

Multiple methods can be used to obtain the food and nutrient intake including a 24-hour recall, food frequency questionnaire, and food records, logs, or diaries.

In the acute care setting, calorie counts are frequently utilized. Unfortunately, calorie counts are not very reliable or efficient as intake is often not recorded or incorrectly recorded. Observation of the patient eating at several meals or taking a 24-hour recall most likely has greater accuracy than calorie counts.

Many advantages and disadvantages have been identified for each method (see Table 3.2) (2–7). The information gathered to determine food and nutrient intake/ history may include qualitative or semiquantitative data. To increase the accuracy of the diet history, multiple methods are often used together.

Table 3.2   Methods for Determining Food and Nutrient Intake

24–hour recall
Method: Food, beverage, and supplement consumption for the past 24 hours provided
Advantages:
- Simple, quick
- Most patients can recall foods eaten
- Reading and writing skills are not required
- Does not influence usual diet patterns

(continued)

Table 3.2   Methods for Determining Food and Nutrient Intake
(continued)

Disadvantages:
- Reliance on patient to accurately recall foods eaten and portion sizes
- Interviewer must interpret portion sizes
- May not be representative of usual intake

Food frequency

Method: Patient selects from a list which foods, beverages, and supplements are frequently consumed

Advantages:
- Can provide an overall evaluation of which nutrients are consumed over time
- Easily standardized
- Beneficial when used with 24–hour recall

Disadvantages:
- Requires patient to remember foods eaten
- Does not give data on daily food portions or meal patterns
- Reading and writing ability required unless patient is interviewed
- Food list may not represent all foods patient eats

Food diary/record

Method: A 3- to 7-day record of all food, beverages, and supplements consumed; should include a weekend day

Advantages:
- Provides data about serving sizes, food preparation method, and time food was eaten
- Reduces error due to reliance on "recall"

Disadvantages:
- Large commitment for the patient
- Requires reading and writing skills
- Process itself may alter normal food consumption patterns
- Recorder must be familiar with portion sizes

(continued)

Table 3.2   Methods for Determining Food and Nutrient Intake
             (continued)

Nutrient intake record (calorie count)

Method: Recording of actual nutrient consumption via direct
observation or tray audit

Advantages:

- Visual observation of actual eating patterns rather than reliance
  on patient interpretation
- Useful for hospitalized or long-term-care facility patients if
  done accurately

Disadvantages:

- Usually subjective estimates of nutrient consumption by
  patient, nurses, family members
- Observers usually poorly trained
- Serving sizes may vary
- Waiting for results is time consuming and may delay optimal
  nutrition intervention
- Low priority and often incomplete
- Frequently inaccurate

Source: Data are from references 2–7.

Questions to Assess Food/Nutrient Intake and History

Tables 3.3 through 3.6 list age-specific food and nutrient
intake/history questions for infants and children, adolescents, older adults, and pregnant women (4,8–11). Some
of the suggested questions are appropriate for other patient
classes as well.

**Table 3.3   Food and Nutrient Intake History Questions for
             Caregivers of Infants and Children**

- What type of milk (eg, breast milk, cow's milk, soy milk,
  rice milk, [note fat content], or formula) are you feeding your
  child?
- How many times per day are you nursing?
- How much water and formula do you use in preparing your
  child's formula?

                                              (continued)

Table 3.3   Food and Nutrient Intake History Questions for Caregivers of Infants and Children (continued)

- How do you prepare formula?
- What water source do you use to prepare formula?
- How many ounces of formula or milk does your child drink each day?
- How many wet diapers does your child have per day?
- What else does your child drink during the day (eg, juice [100%?], soft drinks, tea, water)?
- Do you put your child to bed with a bottle? What's in it?
- What solid foods does your child eat? When were these introduced into their diet?
- How many meals does your child eat per day?
- Does your child snack? If so, how often and what does it consist of?
- Does your child consume sweetened beverages (juice, fruit drinks, soda)? If so, how much?
- Does your child avoid any specific foods or food groups (eg, milk, meats, vegetables)?
- Does your child take any vitamin, mineral, iron, fluoride, or food supplements? If so, how often?
- Does your child ever chew on any nonfood items such as clay, dirt, paint chips, or woodwork?
- How old is your home? Does it have lead pipes or lead paint? Has the water ever been checked for lead? Are you renovating your home?
- How much "screen time" does your child get every day (television, computer, video game, smartphone usage)?

Source: Data are from references 4, 8, and 9.

Table 3.4   Food and Nutrient Intake History Questions for Adolescents

- How many meals do you eat per day?
- Do you skip meals?
- How many meals are eaten away from home each day? Which ones? Where are they obtained?
- Who prepares meals at home?
- Are any specific foods or food groups avoided? Which ones and why?

(continued)

Table 3.4   Food and Nutrient Intake History Questions for Adolescents (continued)

- Do you consume milk or yogurt? What type and how much daily?
- Are you following any special diet? (Evaluate compliance based on diet recall, etc)
- If the teenager has diabetes mellitus, does he or she self-monitor blood glucose levels? How often? What are the results? What are the patient's self-management skills?
- In the past month have you observed any changes in your dietary intake? Your weight?
- Do you drink alcohol? Type (ie, wine, beer, liquor), quantity, frequency, duration?
- Does the teenager exhibit poor self-esteem or body image?
- Have you ever induced vomiting or taken diuretics or cathartics to lose weight or keep from gaining weight?
- Are you physically active? How often do you exercise? What type of exercise do you do? How long do you do the exercise? Are you tired when you finish exercising?
- How much "screen time" do you get every day (television, computer, video game, smartphone usage)?

Source: Data are from references 4, 8, and 9.

Table 3.5   Food and Nutrient Intake History Questions for Older Adults

- Where do you live and with whom?
- Are you physically active? Are you housebound? Describe daily activity.
- Who prepares your meals?
- Who does the food shopping?
- Do you follow any special dietary restrictions? If so, what?
- Do you consume alcohol or use tobacco products? If so, what types, how much, and how frequently?
- Do you take any fiber or food supplements? If so, which ones? How often and what quantity?
- Do you have trouble chewing or swallowing?
- Have you had any changes in bowel habits in the past 2 weeks? If so, how?

(continued)

Table 3.5   Food and Nutrient Intake History Questions for Older Adults (continued)

- Do you avoid any foods or food groups? If so, which ones?
- How much fluid do you drink each day? What do you drink?
- How many meals do you eat per day? How much of each meal do you consume?
- Have you lost or gained weight in the past month without trying?

Source: Data are from references 10 and 11.

Table 3.6   Food and Nutrient Intake History Questions for Pregnant Women

- Did you follow any special diet before pregnancy?
- How much weight have you gained? Are you happy with this weight gain?
- Do you take prenatal vitamins? How often?
- Do you take any iron supplements?
- Do you take calcium supplements?
- Do you have any food allergies? If so, to what?
- Do you have any nonfood cravings (eg, ice, dirt, cornstarch, clay, detergent)?
- Do you drink alcohol? If so, quantity, frequency, and duration?
- How many meals do you eat daily? How many snacks?
- Do you avoid any specific foods, such as fruits, milk or dairy products, vegetables, or meats?
- How much milk or yogurt do you drink/eat, and what type?
- Do you have diabetes? If yes:
  - What type do you have (type 1, type 2, gestational diabetes, prediabetes)?
  - Do you self-monitor your blood glucose levels? If so, what are your glucose levels?
- Do you have a history of gestational diabetes?
- Are you experiencing morning sickness? Feeling nauseated and/or vomiting throughout the day? How often?
- Are you nauseated or vomiting so that you are unable to eat certain foods? If so, which ones?

Source: Data are from reference 10 (reproduction/obstetrics section).

Food and Nutrient Administration

Determination of food and nutrient administration entails collecting information about current and previous diets, the eating environment and how it is affecting intake, and the delivery of enteral and parenteral nutrition. Table 3.7 contains a suggested list of information to gather to determine food and nutrient administration (1).

Table 3.7   Food and Nutrition Administration Components

Current diet order (eg, general, modified, enteral, or parenteral)
Current dietary habits
Days on clear liquids, inadequate intake, or nothing by mouth (NPO)
Dietary restrictions and modifications (past and present)
Recent dietary changes (intentional vs unintentional)
Food consistency modifications (soft, pureed, or liquid)
Appetite assessment (poor, fair, good, or excellent)
Satiety level
Snack consumption
Beverage consumption
Alcohol consumption
Food intolerances
Food allergies
Taste changes or aversions
Ethnic, religious, and cultural dietary influences
Fad diets
Vitamin and mineral supplements
Herbal supplements
Commercial dietary supplements, protein powders, meal replacements, etc
Eating environment (location, atmosphere, companions/assistance)

Source: Data are from reference 1.

Much of the information in Table 3.7 can be found in the patient's medical record. The provider orders section contains information about diets and other nutrition-related orders. Other information, such as problems eating prior to admission, use of over-the-counter medications, or unintentional weight loss or gain might be found in the nursing admission assessment. Socioeconomic information can be located in several places, such as an admission fact sheet, the patient history and physical examination records, and admission assessments done by other services. Because each health care organization may have different policies for documenting information, RDNs should become familiar with procedures used in their workplace.

Medication and Complementary/Alternative Medicine Use

Medications, herbal supplements, other dietary supplements, and other forms of complementary/alternative medicine can play a significant role in nutrient intake and metabolism, as well as overall health (see Chapter 7).

Knowledge/Beliefs/Attitudes

Table 3.8 lists some relevant issues to explore in the assessment of nutrition-related knowledge, beliefs, and attitudes (1). It is possible for nutrition misinformation to impact adequacy of diet; therefore, depending on the goals of the nutrition assessment and intervention, nutrition-related knowledge can be an important area to explore with the patient or client. In general, assessment of knowledge, beliefs, and attitudes lends itself to the outpatient setting, and it may take multiple encounters to determine knowledge gains and changes in beliefs and attitudes.

Table 3.8   Areas of Assessment for Nutrition-Related Knowledge, Beliefs, and Attitudes

Area(s) and level of knowledge/skill
Personal/family value system
Body image
End-of-life decisions
Motivation
Preoccupation with food/nutrients or with weight
Readiness to change behaviors
Self-efficacy
Self-talk/cognitions
Unrealistic goals
Unscientific beliefs/attitudes
Food preferences
Emotions

Source: Data are from reference 1.

Behavior

Nutrition behaviors encompass adherence, avoidance behavior, bingeing and purging behavior, mealtime behavior, and social networks (1). As with knowledge and beliefs, evaluation of nutrition-related behaviors is often most relevant in the outpatient setting with long-term follow-up. However, behaviors and their relationship to the patient's social history (see Chapter 7) should be evaluated if germane, regardless of the setting.

Factors Affecting Access to Food and Food/Nutrition-Related Supplies

Assessing the patient's ability to access food and nutrition-related supplies is essential. For example, if the recommendation is for the patient to follow a special diet after discharge but they are homeless and eat at a shelter, compliance with this recommendation might be impossible. Access to food is also tied to the social history (see Chapter 7) and underscores the importance of looking at patients as individuals with a set of life circumstances instead of as people defined only by their health status or particular medical diagnoses. For more information on food security in the United States, see references 12 and 13.

Physical Activity and Function

Assessment of functional capacity is a vital component of the nutrition assessment (14). For example, the elderly are at high risk for decline in nutritional status if they are unable to perform nutrition-related activities of daily living, such as shopping and preparing food. Hospitalized and long-term care patients who are unable to feed themselves should have a physician's order for assistance with feeding.

The RDN should determine the type, frequency, and intensity of a patient's/client's physical activity. Physical activity level should be evaluated because activity plays a role in the amount of lean body mass (15). Decreased lean body mass is thought to be associated with increased risk for falls, infections, delayed wound healing, and development of pressure ulcers. See reference 16 for a recent review of clinical and research applications in physical activity assessment.

Nutrition-Related Patient/Client-Centered Measures

The patient's nutrition quality of life (QOL) is often tied to their overall well-being (1,17). For example, individuals with gastrointestinal failure who are on long-term nutrition support may find that their inability to enjoy the social aspect of eating has a negative impact on their social life/QOL. RDNs should keep in mind the impact of nutrition interventions on the patient's QOL and strive to find a balance between ideal and realistic goals.

SPECIAL CIRCUMSTANCES

When the patient's capacity to impart their FNRH history is impaired, another person, such as a spouse, child or sibling, will need to act as a surrogate. If no one is present to question, review the medical record to determine whether there is a person that can be contacted by phone to obtain the history. Someone designated as the durable power of attorney or health care proxy is the ideal individual to contact. In cases when the patient is incapacitated and no one else is available for questioning, the clinician will have to rely on other assessment techniques, such as anthropometric measurements and nutrition-focused physical findings, to evaluate the nutritional status of the patient.

REFERENCES

1. Academy of Nutrition and Dietetics. eNCPT: Nutrition Care Process Terminology. 2014. http://ncpt.webauthor.com. Accessed April 15, 2015.
2. Russell MK, Mueller C. Nutrition screening and assessment. In: Gottschlich M, DeLegge M, Mattox T, Mueller C, Worthington P, eds. *The A.S.P.E.N. Nutrition Support Core Curriculum: A Case-Based Approach—The Adult Patient*. Silver Spring, MD: ASPEN; 2007:163–186.
3. Johnson RK. Dietary intake: How do we measure what people are really eating? *Obesity Res*. 2002;10(Suppl 11):63S-68S.
4. Australasian Child and Adolescent Obesity Research Network. Dietary Intake Assessment. www.acaorn.org.au/streams/nutrition/dietary-intake/index.php. Accessed April 15, 2015.
5. Tabacchi G, Amodio E, Di Pasquale M, Bianco A, Jemni M, Mammina C. Validation and reproducibility of dietary assessment methods in adolescents: A systematic literature review. *Public Health Nutr*. 2013;Nov 18:1–15 (Epub ahead of print). www.ncbi.nlm.nih.gov/pubmed/24476625.
6. Samaras D, Samaras N, Bertrand PC, Forster A, Herrmann F, Lesourd B, Lang PO. Comparison of the interobserver variability of two different methods of dietary assessment in a geriatric ward: A pilot study. *J Am Med Dir Assoc*. 2012;13(3):309.e9–e13.

7. Applied Research Cancer Control and Population Sciences. Data Collection Instruments. http://appliedresearch.cancer.gov/resource/collection.html. Accessed April 15, 2015.

8. Food and nutrition history. In: Leonberg BL. *Pocket Guide to Pediatric Nutrition Assessment.* 2nd ed. Chicago, IL: Academy of Nutrition and Dietetics; 2013:93–120.

9. Academy of Nutrition and Dietetics. Pediatric Nutrition Care Manual. www.nutritioncaremanual.org. Accessed April 15, 2015.

10. Academy of Nutrition and Dietetics. Nutrition Care Manual. www.nutritioncaremanual.org. Accessed April 15, 2015.

11. Nutrition assessment. In: Niedert KC, Dorner B, ed. *Nutrition Care of the Older Adult.* 2nd ed. Chicago, IL: American Dietetic Association; 2004:104–133.

12. Hunger in America. Feeding America website. www.feeding america.org/hunger-in-america. Accessed April 15, 2015.

13. US Department of Agriculture Economic Research Service. Food Security in the U.S. www.ers.usda.gov/topics/food-nutrition-assistance/food-security-in-the-us.aspx#.U-t-jPldU4M. Accessed April 15, 2015.

14. White JV. Risk factors for poor nutritional status. *Prim Care.* 1994;21(1):19–31.

15. Bann D, Kuh D, Wills AK, Adams J, Brage S, Cooper R; National Survey of Health and Development scientific and data collection team. Physical activity across adulthood in relation to fat and lean body mass in early old age: Findings from the Medical Research Council National Survey of Health and Development, 1946–2010. *Am J Epidemiol.* 2014;179(10):1197–1207.

16. Strath SJ, Kaminsky LA, Ainsworth BE, Ekelund U, Freedson PS, Gary RA, Richardson CR, Smith DT, Swartz AM; American Heart Association Physical Activity Committee of the Council on Lifestyle and Cardiometabolic Health and Cardiovascular, Exercise, Cardiac Rehabilitation and Prevention Committee of the Council on Clinical Cardiology, and Council. Guide to the assessment of physical activity: Clinical and research applications: A scientific statement from the American Heart Association. *Circulation.* 2013 Nov 12;128(20):2259–79.

17. Carson TL, Hidalgo B, Ard JD, Affuso O. Dietary interventions and quality of life: A systematic review of the literature. *J Nutr Educ Behav.* 2014;46(2):90–101.

Chapter 4

Anthropometric Measurements

Jennifer C. Lefton, MS, RD, LD,
CNSC, FAND

INTRODUCTION

Anthropometric measurements provide clinicians with direct or indirect information about body composition. Height, weight, and changes in weight and growth patterns in infants and children are used to measure body composition and the physical proportions of the body (1). These measurements are useful for evaluating overnutrition and undernutrition as well as monitoring the results of nutrition interventions (2). For example, determination of body composition (eg, fat-free mass) can improve efficacy of nutrition support by allowing the clinician to tailor nutrition therapy and optimize nutritional status.

Accurate anthropometric assessment has the potential to attenuate negative effects of malnutrition, thus improving clinical outcomes and quality of life (3). On the other hand, errors in anthropometric measurement can have far-reaching implications, including errors in medication dosing or in nutrition-related therapies (1).

MEASURING/ESTIMATING HEIGHT

Height and weight are the most commonly used anthropometric measures. Accurate measurement of height is necessary to determine body mass index (BMI), ideal body weight (IBW), or desired body weight (DBW). Actual measurement of height using calibrated equipment is always preferred to a caregiver's or patient's estimations, which do not have an acceptable level of accuracy (4,5). When actual height measurement is not possible, measurement of knee height or arm span may provide reasonable estimations.

Methods for Measuring Height

For an accurate measurement of height, the person measured must be able to stand or lie flat.

Standing Height

To measure standing height, use a measuring rod called a *stadiometer* and the technique described in Table 4.1 (6–8).

Table 4.1   Technique for Measuring Standing Height

1. Choose a place to measure the patient where the floor is firm and even.
2. Ensure that the patient is standing correctly.
   - Feet should be shoeless, with heels close together and touching the wall or stadiometer base.
   - Posture should not be stretched or slumped, with buttocks and back of shoulders touching the stadiometer.
   - Head should not be tipped backward or forward.
   - Eyes should look straight ahead and be in a line parallel to the floor.
3. Move the stadiometer bar to rest gently on the top of the patient's head, compressing hair.
4. Measure height to the nearest 0.1 cm.

Source: Data are from references 6, 7, and 8.

Recumbent Length

To estimate height in a comatose or critically ill patient, recumbent length may be measured with a tape measure while the person is at rest in bed.

Recumbent methods are also used to measure length in infants and children younger than two or three years of age. Refer to the World Health Organization's *Training Course on Child Growth Assessment* (6) for additional guidance on measuring recumbent length in children.

Estimating Height

Nonambulatory individuals and those with contractures, paralysis, or other conditions that limit their ability to stand will require an estimation of their height (9). Arm span and knee height estimation methods may be used in these situations (2).

Arm Span Method

Table 4.2 explains the arm span method (10). Reliable measurements of arm span may be difficult in those individuals with contractures or spinal deformities and in those who are unable to fully extend their arms.

Table 4.2   Arm Span Method for Estimating Height

1. Have the patient extend a straight arm to the side, at a 90-degree angle from the body.
2. Measure the length from the sternal notch to the longest finger on the dominant hand.
3. To estimate height, multiply the arm span measurement by 2.

Source: Data are from reference 10.

Knee Height Method

Knee height measurement, performed with specially designed sliding calipers can be used to estimate height. This method may be appropriate when clients are unable to stand or have excessive spinal curvature. The technique for measuring knee height is described in Table 4.3 (8).

Table 4.3   How to Measure Knee Height

---

1. Take two measurements taken in quick succession:
    a. Begin with the patient in a supine position, with the left leg bent so the knee and ankle are positioned at a 90° angle.
    b. Place the fixed blade of the caliper under the heel and the sliding blade on the anterior thigh, proximal to the patella.
    c. Before reading the caliper measurement, apply pressure to compress the tissue.
    d. Measurements should be within 0.5 cm of each other.
2. Calculate the mean of the two measurements. To estimate height from knee height, use this mean and the appropriate formula for the patient based on age, ethnicity/race, and sex (see Tables 4.4 and 4.5).

In 1985 Chumlea et al used a small sample of non-Hispanic whites to develop equations for use in the elderly population (11). Further research concluded that these equations did not accurately predict height across all ethnic groups (12).

Subsequently, Chumlea and colleagues used nationally representative data to publish new equations for black and white Americans between the ages of 6 and 60 years (13) and non-Hispanic white, non-Hispanic black, and Mexican-American individuals older than 60 years (14). These equations are presented in Tables 4.4 and 4.5 (13,14). Additional population-specific formulas for elderly patients can be found in Appendix 2 of reference 8.

Table 4.4 Selected Equations for Estimating Height from Knee Height in Males[a]

Population	Equation to Estimate Height	SEI
Ages 6–17 y		
Blacks	$39.60 + (2.18 \times \text{Knee Height})$	4.58
Whites	$40.54 + (2.22 \times \text{Knee Height})$	4.21
Ages 18–60 y		
Blacks	$73.42 + (1.79 \times \text{Knee Height})$	3.6
Whites	$71.85 + (1.88 \times \text{Knee Height})$	3.97
Age > 60 y		
Non-Hispanic blacks	$79.69 + (1.85 \times \text{Knee Height}) - (0.14 \times \text{Age})$	3.81
Non-Hispanic whites	$78.31 + (1.94 \times \text{Knee Height}) - (0.14 \times \text{Age})$	3.74
Mexican-Americans	$82.77 + (1.83 \times \text{Knee Height}) - (0.16 \times \text{Age})$	3.69

[a]Where: Knee height and standard error for an individual (SEI) are measured in cm, and age is measured in years.
Source: Data are from references 13 and 14.

Table 4.5 Selected Equations for Estimating Height from Knee Height in Females[a]

Population	Equation to Estimate Height	SEI
Ages 6–17 y		
Blacks	$46.59 + (2.02 \times \text{Knee Height})$	4.39
Whites	$43.21 + (2.15 \times \text{Knee Height})$	3.9
Ages 18–60 y		
Blacks	$68.10 + (1.86 \times \text{Knee Height}) - (0.06 \times \text{Age})$	3.8
Whites	$70.25 + (1.87 \times \text{Knee Height}) - (0.06 \times \text{Age})$	3.6

(continued)

Table 4.5 Selected Equations for Estimating Height from Knee Height in Females^a (continued)

Population	Equation to Estimate Height	SEI
Ages > 60 y		
Non-Hispanic blacks	89.58 + (1.61 × Knee Height) – (0.17 × Age)	3.83
Non-Hispanic whites	82.21 + (1.85 × Knee Height) – (0.21 × Age)	3.98
Mexican-Americans	84.25 + (1.82 × Knee Height) – (0.26 × Age)	3.78

^{a}Where: Knee height and standard error for an individual (SEI) are measured in cm, and age is measured in years.
Source: Data are from references 13 and 14.

MEASURING WEIGHT

To effectively use weight in the assessment of a client/patient's nutritional status, it is important to obtain accurate measurements, using calibrated equipment, and document weight changes over time (eg, weight at admission or start of intervention, current weight, and usual body weight [UBW]) (2). Patient recall should not be relied on for the weight history.

Scales used to determine body weight must be regularly calibrated, particularly if they are used frequently.

- Spring scales, the type seen in most bathroom scales, are least accurate.
- Beam and balance scales, the types frequently seen in provider offices, have a higher degree of accuracy.
- Electronic scales are most accurate. In some care settings, it is possible to interface electronic scales with the electronic medical record so the measurements are immediately entered into the medical record.

Regardless of the type of scale used, measurement accuracy requires that the patient have the ability to stand/sit still for the few seconds required for measurement. This is often difficult when weighing infants and small children. Accuracy is improved by taking three or four measurements and finding the average (if the measurements are reasonably similar) or by first weighing infant/child's caregiver and then weighing the caregiver while holding the infant/child and subtracting the weight of the caregiver.

Hospital scales can include various types, including standing and sitting scales, a lift scale, or a bed scale. All types of scales other than an actual bed scale must be calibrated by the hospital biomedical technicians. Bed scale calibration is often performed by the bedside nurse and is an important step prior to measuring the patient's weight. Inaccuracies can occur if additional items are included in the bed while the patient's weight is obtained.

BODY MASS INDEX

Body mass index (BMI) is a ratio of weight to height and is used as an estimate of body fat in the healthy population.

Equations

BMI can be calculated using the equations in Table 4.6.

Table 4.6   Calculating Body Mass Index (BMI)

Measurement System	Equation
Metric	Weight (kg)/Height (m^2)
English	[Weight (lb)/Height (in)^2] × 703.1

Interpretation

Nomograms and charts are available for interpretation of BMI (15). BMI is considered to be an estimation of overnutrition or undernutrition and is used to evaluate adiposity (see Table 4.7) (16,17).

Table 4.7   **Body Mass Index (BMI)
Classification in Adults**

BMI	Classification
≥40	Obesity grade III
35–39.9	Obesity grade II
30–34.9	Obesity grade I
25–29.9	Overweight
18.5–24.9	Normal
<18.5	Underweight
17–18.4	Mild thinness
16–16.9	Moderate thinness
<16	Severe thinness

Source: Data are from references 16 and 17.

Although BMI does not measure body fat directly, many researchers and practitioners think that it provides an acceptable estimation of body fat. However, recent research comparing BMI to bioelectric impedance in healthy adults found that BMI did not correlate well to the percentage of body fat measured by bioelectric impedance (18). As with any other diagnostic tool, BMI should be evaluated in conjunction with other information related to the patient's health status.

Pediatric Populations

In pediatric populations, BMI is interpreted through the use of age- and sex-specific percentiles or *z* scores. Refer to the World Health Organization for children birth to two years (http://www.who.int/childgrowth/standards /weight_for_age/en/), refer to Centers for Disease Control and Prevention for patients aged 2–20 years (www.cdec .gov/growthchats), and refer to Leonberg (19) for additional information on the use of BMI for evaluation of pediatric patients.

Acutely Ill Patients

The use of BMI has not been validated in acutely ill patients. However, BMI is frequently used in the assessment of acutely ill patients and may be one of several potential indicators leading to a nutrition diagnosis (20).

BMI Data in Electronic Medical Records

Most electronic medical records automatically calculate BMI based on the height and weight data entered on admission. It is important to carefully evaluate admission BMI, noting whether stated or estimated height and weight were used for the initial BMI calculations. Results must be interpreted individually.

Additional Considerations

The correlation between BMI and body fatness is less accurate in those with an increased percentage of fat-free mass (eg, athletes), an increased percentage of fat mass (eg, patients with spinal cord injuries), or with fluid imbalances (eg, edema).

Additionally, mortality is not increased in older adults with a BMI result that is considered overweight, and some contend that the normal weight BMI range may be too restrictive when used for the elderly (21,22).

IDEAL BODY WEIGHT

There is no consensus about the definition of "ideal" or "desirable" body weight and, consequently, it is not possible to identify a single estimation method that is most accurate/valid (23). It may be more clinically relevant in acute care to compare the patient's current weight to their typical or usual body weight.

Actuarial Tables

Historically, height-weight tables have defined IBW or desirable body weight as the weight associated with the lowest mortality determined by actuarial data from life insurance companies (24–26). The 1983 Metropolitan tables determined IBW based on height and body frame size, which was obtained by determining elbow breadth measurements (27).

Ideal Body Weight Based on Body Mass Index

As shown in Table 4.8, an individual's BMI and height can be used to calculate the weight range that would be within the "normal BMI" range. Shah et al (28) suggest that it may be useful to compare other methods of estimating IBW to the weight that corresponds to a BMI of 22. Various IBW calculators choose other BMI values within the normal range as the basis for determining an IBW. Refer to the previous section of this chapter for information on the potential limitations of BMI for evaluating adiposity.

Table 4.8   Calculating Weight Range Within Normal Body Mass Index (BMI) Range

Method
1. Determine the individual's height.
2. Use the height and the lower and upper ends of the normal BMI range (18.5–24.9) to find the lower and upper ends of the weight range:

Lower End of Weight Range (kg) = $18.5 \times$ Height (m^2)

Upper End of Weight Range (kg) = $24.9 \times$ Height (m^2)

Example
Calculate the normal weight range for a man who is 6 feet, 3 inches (1.9 meters) tall:

Lower end of weight range = $18.5 \times 1.9 \times 1.9 = 66.8$ kg

Upper end of weight range = $24.9 \times 1.9 \times 1.9 = 89.9$ kg

Hamwi Formula

The Hamwi formula (Table 4.9) (29) is frequently used by health care workers in clinical situations to estimate IBW.

Table 4.9 Estimating Ideal Body Weight (IBW) with the Hamwi Formula

Equation for men

IBW (lb) = 106 lb for the first 5 feet plus 6 lb for every inch thereafter

IBW (kg) = 48.08 kg for the first 152 cm plus 1.07 kg for every centimeter thereafter

Equation for women

IBW (lb) = 100 lb for the first 5 feet plus 5 lb for every inch thereafter

IBW (kg) = 45.35 kg for the first 152 cm plus 0.89 kg for every centimeter thereafter

Example

Calculate IBW for a man who is 6 feet, 3 inches tall (15 inches more than 5 feet)/1.90 meters (38 cm more than 152 cm):

$$IBW = 106 + (6 \times 15) = 106 + 90 = 196 \text{ lb}$$

$$IBW = 48.08 + (1.07 \times 38) = 48.08 + 40.66 = 88.76 \text{ kg}$$

Source: Equations are from reference 29.

Adjustments for body frame size are sometimes made when estimating the IBW. For both metric and standard formulas, 10% can be added or subtracted to the final value to accommodate variations in body frame size.

Other IBW Formulas

The Devine formula (Table 4.10) (30) was originally intended to be used in calculating medication dosages and is now employed in some online IBW calculators. Another equation that is sometimes used in IBW calculators is the Robinson formula (Table 4.11) (31).

Table 4.10   Estimating Ideal Body Weight (IBW) with the Devine Formula

Equation for men

> IBW (kg) = 50 kg for the first 5 feet + 2.3 kg for every inch thereafter

Equation for women

> IBW (kg) = 45.5 kg for the first 5 feet + 2.3 kg for every inch thereafter

Example

Calculate IBW for a man who is 6 feet, 3 inches tall (15 inches more than 5 feet).

> IBW = 50 + (2.3 × 15) = 50 + 34.5 = 84.5 kg

Source: Equations are from reference 30.

Table 4.11   Estimating Ideal Body Weight (IBW) with the Robinson Formula

Equation for men

> IBW (kg) = 52 kg for the first 5 feet + 1.9 kg for every inch thereafter

Equation for women

> IBW (kg) = 49 kg for the first 5 feet + 1.7 kg for every inch thereafter

Example

Calculate IBW for a man who is 6 feet, 3 inches tall (15 inches more than 5 feet).

> IBW = 52 + (1.9 × 15) = 52 + 28.5 = 80.5 kg

Source: Equations are from reference 31.

Adjustments to IBW for Obesity

Adjustment of ideal body weight to establish the nutrient prescription in obese patients is controversial and should not be used. There is no strong evidence supporting such adjustments. Refer to your pharmacy practitioner for use of adjusted IBW in medication prescription and dosing.

Adjustments to IBW for Spinal Cord Injury

Assessment of patients with spinal cord injury is impacted by loss of muscle function due to paralysis. According to the Academy of Nutrition and Dietetics Evidence-Based Nutrition Practice Guideline for Spinal Cord Injury (32), IBW should be estimated by adjusting the Metropolitan Life Insurance tables for individuals of equivalent height and weight. There are two reported methods for adjusting the tables (32):

- Method 1:
  - Quadriplegia: Reduction of 10% to 15% lower than table weight
  - Paraplegia: Reduction of 5% to 10% lower than table weight
- Method 2:
  - Quadriplegia: 15 to 20 lb lower than table weight
  - Paraplegia: 10 to 15 lb lower than table weight

Adjustments to IBW for Amputated Body Components

If amputation has occurred, estimation of the IBW must be adjusted to account for the missing parts (see Table 4.12). The formula used to make this estimate is based on the percentage of body weight contributed by the specific body parts (33).

Table 4.12   Adjusting Ideal Body Weight (IBW) for Amputation

Equation

$$\text{Adjusted IBW} = \frac{100\% - \% \text{ Amputation}}{100\%} \times \text{IBW for Original Height}$$

Percentage of body weight contributed by specific body parts

- Trunk w/o limbs: 50%
- Hand: 0.7%
- Forearm with hand: 2.3%
- Forearm without hand: 1.6%
- Upper arm: 2.7%
- Entire arm: 5%
- Foot: 1.5%
- Lower leg with foot: 5.9%
- Lower leg without foot: 4.4%
- Thigh: 10.1%
- Entire leg: 16%

Example

Calculated adjusted IBW for a patient (original IBW 166 lb) who has had a below-the-knee amputation (lower leg with foot = 5.9% of body weight).

$$\text{Adjusted IBW} = \frac{100\% - 5.9\%}{100\%} \times 166 \text{ lb}$$

$$\text{Adjusted IBW} = \frac{94.1\%}{100\%} \times 166 = 0.941 \times 166 = 156 \text{ lb}$$

Source: Data are from reference 33.

INTERPRETATION OF BODY WEIGHT

Body weight is affected by fluid shifts, disease state, treatment, and inflammatory state. (9). When evaluating weight as an indicator of a client's/patient's nutritional status, it can be helpful to calculate the percentage of weight change over time (the weight pattern) (2).

The significance of the percentage of weight change depends on the length of time in which the weight change occurred, as well as whether the weight loss was intentional or unintentional (see Table 4.13) (34).

Table 4.13   Assessing Percentage of Weight Change

Equation

$$\% \text{ Weight Change} = \frac{\text{UBW} - \text{CBW}}{\text{UBW}} \times 100$$

Interpretation

	Percentage of Weight Change	
Time Frame	Significant Weight Loss	Severe Weight Loss
1 wk	1%–2%	>2%
1 mo	5%	>5%
3 mo	7.5%	>7.5%
6 mo	10%	>10%

Example

Calculate % weight change for a patient whose weight decreases from 129 lb to 101 lb in 6 months.

$$\% \text{ Weight Change} = \frac{129 \text{ lb} - 101 \text{ lb}}{129 \text{ lb}} \times 100$$

$$\% \text{ Weight Change} = \frac{28 \text{ lb}}{129 \text{ lb}} = 0.22 \times 100 = 22\% \text{ (severe weight loss)}$$

Source: Data are from reference 34.

BODY COMPOSITION

Measurement of body weight provides a one-dimensional view of body composition. Variation in fat-free mass (FFM), skeletal size, and adiposity can contribute to differences in body weight between individuals of the same height (2).

Thibault and Pichard (35) propose that because obesity and chronic disease are often comorbid conditions, there is increased risk of underestimation of FFM loss in obese patients. Evaluation of weight loss and interpretation of BMI are not adequately sensitive to detect the loss of lean body mass. For example, a high BMI could disguise significant loss of FFM at hospital admission.

Clinicians have long believed that FFM loss is likely associated with decreased survival, a worse clinical outcome, decreased quality of life, and increased health care costs. Accurate body composition evaluation for hospitalized and critically ill patients could help clinicians assess nutritional status accurately.

Indirect Methods for Measuring Body Composition

Indirect methods used in the measurement of body composition include triceps skinfold (TSF), an index of body fat stores; and midarm muscle circumference (MAMC) and midarm circumference (MAC), both of which represent muscle protein (9). These measures have limited validity in the acute-care setting for the following reasons:

- Clinicians performing measurements may be inexperienced
- Alterations in the patient's fluid status
- Variation in body composition in selected populations (eg, athletes, individuals with spinal cord injuries)
- Lack of appropriate standards for acutely ill populations

Derived Parameters

Derived anthropometric parameters include arm muscle area (AMA) and mid-upper arm fat area (AFA). AFA and AMA are based on measurements of TSF and midarm circumference (MAC).

Calculations

Table 4.14 provides four equations to correct for bone area that are used to allow a more accurate assessment of bone-free muscle area (36).

Table 4.14   Calculating Total Upper Arm Area, Uncorrected and Corrected Arm Muscle Area, and Mid-Upper Arm Fat Area

Total upper arm area equation

$$TAA \ (cm^2) = \frac{MAC \ (cm)^2}{4 \times 3.14}$$

Uncorrected arm muscle area equation

$$AMA \ (cm^2) = \frac{\{MAC \ (cm) - [TSF \ (cm) \times 3.14]\}^2}{4 \times 3.14}$$

Corrected AMA equations

Males: $AMAc \ (cm^2) = AMA \ (cm^2) - 10 \ cm^2$

Females: $AMAc \ (cm^2) = AMA \ (cm^2) - 6.5 \ cm^2$

Mid-upper arm fat area equation

$$AFA \ (cm^2) = TAA \ (cm^2) - AMA \ (cm^2)$$

Examples

1. Calculation of TAA for individual with MAC of 30 cm:

$$TAA = \frac{(30)^2}{4 \times 3.14} = 71.6 \ cm^2$$

2. Calculation of uncorrected AMA for individual with MAC of 30 cm and TSF of 25 mm (2.5 cm):

$$AMA = \frac{[30 - (2.5 \times 3.14)]^2}{4 \times 3.14} = \frac{490.62}{12.56} = 39.1 \ cm^2$$

(continued)

Table 4.14 **Calculating Total Upper Arm Area, Uncorrected and Corrected Arm Muscle Area, and Mid-Upper Arm Fat Area** (continued)

3a. Calculation of corrected AMA for man with AMA of 39.1 cm²:

$$AMAc = 39.1 - 10 = 29.1 \text{ cm}^2$$

3b. Calculation of corrected AMA for woman with AMA of 39 cm²:

$$AMAc = 39.1 - 6.5 = 32.4 \text{ cm}^2$$

4. Calculation of AFA for individual with TAA of 71.6 cm² and AMA of 39.1 cm²:

$$AFA = 71.6 - 39.1 = 32.5 \text{ cm}^2$$

Abbreviations: TAA, total upper arm area; MAC, midarm circumference; TSF, triceps skinfold; AMA, arm muscle area; AMAc, corrected arm muscle area; AFA, upper arm fat area.
Source: Equations are from reference 35.

Interpretation of AFA and AMA

After they are calculated, AFA and AMA are then compared with reference data, measured in mm² (1 cm² = 100 mm²), to determine a percentile rank (37). The reference data (Tables 4.15–4.18) represent measurements obtained from samples from noninstitutionalized adults in the First and Second National Health and Nutrition Examination Surveys (NHANES 1 and NHANES 2). Because the sample used to determine the standards did not include all ethnic groups, the interpretations of AFA and AMA measurements may not be universally valid (37). Performing serial measurements of body composition may be useful for assessing long-term changes in fat mass and fat-free mass. See Table 4.19 for the interpretations of arm muscle and fat areas reflecting alterations in total body weight (38).

Table 4.15 Arm Muscle Area (AMA) Percentiles for Males

Age Group, y	AMA Percentiles, mm²						
	5	10	25	50	75	90	95
1–1.9	956	1014	1133	1278	1447	1644	1720
2–2.9	973	1040	1190	1345	1557	1690	1787
3–3.9	1095	1201	1357	1484	1618	1750	1853
4–4.9	1207	1264	1408	1579	1747	1926	2008
5–5.9	1298	1411	1550	1720	1884	2089	2285
6–6.9	1360	1447	1605	1815	2056	2297	2493
7–7.9	1497	1548	1808	2027	2246	2494	2886
8–8.9	1550	1664	1895	2089	2296	2628	2788
9–9.9	1811	1884	2067	2288	2657	3053	3257
10–10.9	1930	2027	2182	2575	2903	3486	3882
11–11.9	2016	2156	2382	2670	3022	3359	4226
12–12.9	2216	2339	2649	3022	3496	3968	4640
13–13.9	2363	2546	3044	3553	4081	4502	4794
14–14.9	2830	3147	3586	3963	4575	5368	5530
15–15.9	3138	3317	3788	4481	5134	5631	5900
16–16.9	3625	4044	4352	4951	5753	6576	6980
17–17.9	3998	4252	4777	5286	5950	6886	7726
18–18.9	4070	4481	5066	5552	6374	7067	8355
19–24.9	4508	4777	5274	5913	6660	7606	8200
25–34.9	4694	4963	5541	6214	7067	7847	8436
35–44.9	4844	5181	5740	6490	7265	8034	8488
45–54.9	4546	4946	5589	6297	7142	7918	8458
55–64.9	4422	4783	5381	6144	6919	7670	8149
65–74.9	3973	4411	5031	5716	6432	7074	7453

Source: Adapted with permission from reference 37: Frisancho AR. New norms of upper limb fat and muscle areas for assessment of nutritional status. *Am J Clin Nutr.* 1981;34:2540–2545. Copyright American Society for Nutrition.

Table 4.16   Arm Muscle Area (AMA) Percentiles for Females

Age Group, y	AMA Percentiles, mm^2						
	5	10	25	50	75	90	95
1–1.9	885	973	1084	1221	1378	1535	1621
2–2.9	973	1029	1119	1269	1405	1595	1727
3–3.9	1014	1133	1227	1396	1563	1690	1846
4–4.9	1058	1171	1313	1475	1644	1832	1958
5–5.9	1238	1301	1423	1598	1825	2012	2159
6–6.9	1354	1414	1513	1683	1877	2182	2323
7–7.9	1330	1441	1602	1815	2045	2332	2469
8–8.9	1513	1566	1808	2034	2327	2657	2996
9–9.9	1723	1788	1976	2227	2571	2987	3112
10–10.9	1740	1784	2019	2296	2583	2873	3093
11–11.9	1784	1987	2316	2612	3071	3739	3953
12–12.9	2092	2182	2579	2904	3225	3655	3847
13–13.9	2269	2426	2657	3130	3529	4081	4568
14–14.9	2418	2562	2874	3220	3704	4294	4850
15–15.9	2426	2518	2847	3248	3689	4123	4756
16–16.9	2308	2567	2865	3248	3718	4353	4946
17–17.9	2442	2674	2996	3336	3883	4552	5251
18–18.9	2398	2538	2917	3243	3694	4461	4767
19–24.9	2538	2728	3026	3406	3877	4439	4940
25–34.9	2661	2826	3148	3573	4138	4806	5541
35–44.9	2750	2948	3359	3783	4428	5240	5877
45–54.9	2784	2956	3378	3858	4520	5375	5964
55–64.9	2784	3063	3477	4045	4750	5632	6247
65–74.9	2737	3018	3444	4019	4739	5566	6214

Source: Adapted with permission from reference 37: Frisancho AR. New norms of upper limb fat and muscle areas for assessment of nutritional status. *Am J Clin Nutr*. 1981;34:2540–2545. Copyright American Society for Nutrition.

Table 4.17   Arm Fat Area (AFA) Percentiles for Males

Age Group, y	Arm Fat Area Percentiles, mm^2						
	5	10	25	50	75	90	95
1–1.9	452	486	590	741	895	1036	1176
2–2.9	434	504	578	737	871	1044	1148
3–3.9	464	519	590	736	868	1071	1151
4–4.9	428	494	598	722	859	989	1085
5–5.9	446	488	582	713	914	1176	1299
6–6.9	371	446	539	678	896	1115	1519
7–7.9	423	473	574	758	1011	1393	1511
8–8.9	410	460	588	725	1003	1248	1558
9–9.9	485	527	635	859	1252	1864	2081
10–10.9	523	543	738	982	1376	1906	2609
11–11.9	536	595	754	1148	1710	2348	2574
12–12.9	554	650	874	1172	1558	2536	3580
13–13.9	475	570	812	1096	1702	2744	3322
14–14.9	453	563	786	1082	1608	2746	3508
15–15.9	521	595	690	931	1423	2434	3100
16–16.9	542	593	844	1078	1746	2280	3041
17–17.9	598	698	827	1096	1636	2407	2888
18–18.9	560	665	860	1264	1947	3302	3928
19–24.9	594	743	963	1406	2231	3098	3652
25–34.9	675	831	1174	1752	2459	3246	3786
35–44.9	703	851	1310	1792	2463	3098	3624
45–54.9	749	922	1254	1741	2359	3245	3928
55–64.9	658	839	1166	1645	2236	2976	3466
65–74.9	573	753	1122	1621	2199	2876	3327

Source: Adapted with permission from reference 37: Frisancho AR. New norms of upper limb fat and muscle areas for assessment of nutritional status. *Am J Clin Nutr.* 1981;34:2540–2545. Copyright American Society for Nutrition.

Table 4.18   Arm Fat Area (AFA) Percentiles for Females

Age Group, y	Arm Fat Area Percentiles, mm²						
	5	10	25	50	75	90	95
1–1.9	401	466	578	706	847	1022	1140
2–2.9	469	526	642	747	894	1061	1173
3–3.9	473	529	656	822	967	1106	1158
4–4.9	490	541	654	766	907	1109	1236
5–5.9	470	529	647	812	991	1330	1536
6–6.9	464	508	638	827	1009	1263	1436
7–7.9	491	560	706	920	1135	1407	1644
8–8.9	527	634	769	1042	1383	1872	2482
9–9.9	642	690	933	1219	1584	2171	2524
10–10.9	616	702	842	1141	1608	2500	3005
11–11.9	707	802	1015	1301	1942	2730	3690
12–12.9	782	854	1090	1511	2056	2666	3369
13–13.9	726	838	1219	1625	2374	3272	4150
14–14.9	981	1043	1423	1818	2403	3250	3765
15–15.9	839	1126	1396	1886	2544	3093	4195
16–16.9	1126	1351	1663	2006	2598	3374	4236
17–17.9	1042	1267	1463	2104	2977	3864	5159
18–18.9	1003	1230	1616	2104	2617	3508	3733
19–24.9	1046	1198	1596	2166	2959	4050	4896
25–34.9	1173	1399	1841	2548	3512	4690	5560
35–44.9	1336	1619	2158	2898	3932	5093	5847
45–54.9	1459	1803	2447	3244	4229	5416	6140
55–64.9	1345	1879	2520	3369	4360	5276	6152
65–74.9	1363	1681	2266	3063	3943	4914	5530

Source: Adapted with permission from reference 37: Frisancho AR. New norms of upper limb fat and muscle areas for assessment of nutritional status. *Am J Clin Nutr.* 1981;34:2540–2545. Copyright American Society for Nutrition.

**Table 4.19   Arm Muscle and Arm Fat Areas Reflecting
                Alterations in Total Body Weight**

Percentile Rank	AMA	AFA	Total Body Weight
≤5	Muscle deficit	Fat deficit	Total body wasting
5.1–15	Below average	Below average	Below average
15.1–85	Average	Average	Average
>85	Above-average musculature	Excess fat	Excess total body weight

Abbreviations: AMA, arm muscle area; AFA, Mid-upper arm fat area.
Source: Data are from reference 34.

Other Tools for Assessing Body Composition

Other methods for analysis of body composition have
been developed, including dual-energy X-ray absorptiometry (DXA), bioelectrical impedance analysis (BIA),
and computerized tomography (CT). All are too expensive
or cumbersome to be considered in routine assessment of
body composition.

- DXA is a noninvasive method of direct measurement
  of the three components of body composition, however, expensive equipment and cumbersome techniques limit its usefulness in clinical settings.
- BIA is simple and inexpensive and can be used at
  the bedside to evaluate FFM and total body water.
  However, its usefulness in critical illness may be
  limited because FFM can be significantly altered by
  the increase in extracellular water commonly seen in
  critical care patients.
- Targeted CT imaging, common in the management
  of critical care patients, could be used to estimate
  body composition as well, but this method lacks validation (35).

REFERENCES

1. Charney P. Nutrition screening and assessment. In: Skipper A, ed. *Dietitian's Handbook of Enteral and Parenteral Nutrition.* Sudbury, MA: Jones & Bartlett Learning; 2012:4–21.

2. Mahan LK, Raymond JL, eds. *Krause's Food & the Nutrition Care Process.* 13th ed. St Louis, MO: Elsevier; 2012.

3. Thibault R, Genton L, Pichard C. Body composition: Why, when and for who? *Clin Nutr.* 2012;31(4):435–447.

4. Beghetto MG, Fink J, Luft VC, de Mello ED. Estimates of body height in adult patients. *Clin Nutr.* 2006;25(3):438–443.

5. Bloomfield R, Steel E, MacLennan G, Noble DW. Accuracy of weight and height estimation in an intensive care unit: Implications for clinical practice and research. *Crit Care Med.* 2006;34(8):2153–2157.

6. World Health Organization. Training Course on Child Growth Assessment: WHO Growth Standards—Measuring a Child's Growth. 2008. www.who.int/childgrowth/training/module_b _measuring_growth.pdf. Accessed April 15, 2015.

7. Centers for Disease Control and Prevention. About BMI for Children and Teens: Measuring Children's Height and Weight Accurately at Home. www.cdc.gov/healthyweight/assessing /bmi/childrens_bmi/measuring_children.html. Accessed April 15, 2015.

8. Nestlé Nutrition Institute. Nutrition Screening as Easy as MNA. www.mna-elderly.com/forms/mna_guide_english_sf.pdf. Accessed April 15, 2015.

9. Jensen GL, Hsiao PY, Wheeler D. Nutrition screening and assessment. In: Gottschlich MM, ed. *The A.S.P.E.N. Nutrition Support Core Curriculum: A Case-Based Approach—The Adult Patient.* Silver Spring, MD: American Society for Parenteral and Enteral Nutrition; 2012:15–169.

10. Mitchell CO, Lipschitz DA. Arm length measurement as an alternative to height in the nutritional assessment of the elderly. *JPEN J Parenter Enteral Nutr.* 1982;6:226–229.

11. Chumlea WC, Roche AF, Steinbaugh ML. Estimating stature from knee height for persons 60 to 90 years of age. *J Am Geriatr Soc.* 1985;33:116–120.

12. Bermudez OI, Becker EK, Tucker KL. Development of sex-specific equations for estimating stature of frail elderly Hispanics living in the northeastern United States. *Am J Clin Nutr.* 1999;69(5):992–998.

13. Chumlea W, Guo SG, Steinbaugh ML. Prediction of stature from knee height for black and white adults and children with application to mobility-impaired or handicapped persons. *J Am Diet Assoc.* 1994;94(12):1385–1391.

14. Chumlea W, Guo SS, Wholihan K, Cockram D, Kuczmarski RJ, Johnson CL. Stature prediction equations for elderly non-Hispanic white, non-Hispanic black, and Mexican-American persons developed from NHANES III data. *J Am Diet Assoc.* 1998;98(2):137–142.

15. National Heart, Lung, and Blood Institute. Body Mass Index Tables. www.nhlbi.nih.gov/health/educational/lose_wt/BMI /bmi_tbl.htm. Accessed April 15, 2015.

16. Obesity Education Initiative Task Force. *Clinical Guidelines on the Identification, Evaluation, and Treatment of Overweight and Obesity in Adults.* Washington, DC: National Institutes of Health; 1998.

17. World Health Organization. BMI Classification. http://apps .who.int/bmi/index.jsp?introPage=intro_3.html&. Accessed April 15, 2015.

18. Meeuwsen S, Horgan GW, Elia M. The relationship between BMI and percent body fat, measured by bioelectrical impedance, in a large adult sample is curvilinear and influenced by age and sex. *Clin Nutr.* 2010;29(5):560–566.

19. Leonberg BL. *Academy of Nutrition and Dietetics Pocket Guide to Pediatric Nutrition Assessment.* 2nd ed. Chicago, IL: Academy of Nutrition and Dietetics; 2013.

20. Academy of Nutrition and Dietetics. eNCPT: Nutrition Care Process Terminology. 2014. http://ncpt.webauthor.com. Accessed April 15, 2015.

21. Heiat A, Vaccarino V, Krumholz HM. An evidence-based assessment of federal guidelines for overweight and obesity as they apply to elderly patients. *Arch Intern Med.* 2001;161:1194–1203.

22. Winter JE, MacInnis RJ, Wattanapenpaiboon N, Nowson, CA. BMI and all-cause mortality in older adults: A meta-analysis. *Am J Clin Nutr.* ePub ahead of print Jan 22, 2014; doi:10.3945.

23. Academy of Nutrition and Dietetics Evidence Analysis Library. Chronic Kidney Disease Evidence-Based Nutrition Practice Guideline: Use Published Weight Norms with Caution. 2010. www.andeal.org/topic.cfm?menu=5303&cat=3929. Accessed April 15, 2015.

24. Metropolitan Life Insurance Company. Ideal weights for men. *Stat Bull Metropolitan Life Insurance Company.* 1942;23:6–8.

25. Metropolitan Life Insurance Company. Ideal weights for women. *Stat Bull Metropolitan Life Insurance Company*. 1943;24:6–8.

26. Metropolitan Life Insurance Company. New weight standards for men and women. *Stat Bull Metropolitan Life Insurance Company.* 1959;40:1–4.

27. Metropolitan Life Insurance Company. 1983 Metropolitan height and weight tables: New York. *Stat Bull Metropolitan Life Insurance Company.* 1983;64:1–9.

28. Shah B, Sucher K, Hollenbeck CB. Comparison of ideal body weight equations and published height-weight tables with body mass index tables for healthy adults in the United States. *Nutr Clin Pract.* 2006;3:312–319.

29. Hamwi GJ. Changing dietary concepts. In: Donowski TS, ed. *Diabetes Mellitus: Diagnosis and Treatment.* New York, NY: American Diabetes Association; 1964:73–78.

30. Devine BJ. Gentamicin therapy. *Drug Intell Clin Pharm.* 1974;8:650–655.

31. Robinson JD, Lupkiewicz SM, Lopez LM, Ariet M. Determination of ideal body weight for drug dosage calculations. *Am J Hosp Pharm.* 1983;40:1016–1019.

32. Academy of Nutrition and Dietetics. Spinal Cord Injury Evidence-Based Nutrition Practice Guideline. 2009. www.andeal.org/topic.cfm?menu=5292&cat=3485. Accessed April 15, 2015.

33. Osterkamp LK. Current perspective on assessment of human body proportions of relevance to amputees. *J Am Diet Assoc.* 1995;95:215–218.

34. White J, Guenter P, Jensen G. Consensus Statement of the Academy of Nutrition and Dietetics/American Society for Parenteral and Enteral Nutrition: Characteristics recommended for the identification and documentation of adult malnutrition (undernutrition). *J Acad Nutr Diet.* 2012;112:730–738.

35. Thibault R, Pichard C. The evaluation of body composition: A useful tool for clinical practice. *Ann Nutr Metab.* 2012;60:6–16.

36. Howell WH. Anthropometry and body composition analysis. In: Gottschlich MM, Matarese LE, eds. *Contemporary Nutrition Support Practice: A Clinical Guide.* 2nd ed. Philadelphia, PA: WB Saunders; 2003:31–44.

37. Frisancho AR. New norms of upper limb fat and muscle areas for assessment of nutritional status. *Am J Clin Nutr.* 1981;34:2540–2545.

38. Frisancho AR. *Anthropometric Standards for the Assessment of Growth and Nutritional Status.* Ann Arbor, MI: University of Michigan Press; 1990.

Chapter 5

Nutrition-Focused Physical Assessment

Sarah Peterson, MS, RD, CNSC

INTRODUCTION

The information obtained during a physical examination is a fundamental part of a comprehensive nutrition assessment. A nutrition-focused physical assessment combines data from the physical examination, vital signs, and anthropometrics with the information gathered from the patient's medical record, tests, procedures, and laboratory data, and from his or her food-related history and nutrition-related history to determine the optimal nutrition care plan (1–11).

Registered dietitian nutritionists (RDNs) are uniquely trained to evaluate physical examination data to correctly evaluate nutrient-specific physical findings and analyze the role of nutritional status in health maintenance as well as recovery from injury or disease. In the hospital setting, physical assessment is used to evaluate patients for malnutrition, and RDNs must aim to identify loss of muscle or fat mass, decreased functional status, poor oral intake, and increased body weight due to inflammation related fluid accumulation (12–13).

Historically, isolated nutrient deficiencies were rarely identified; however, more recently, they have been reported with increasing frequency (14). In this context, a nutrition-focused physical assessment is essential to identify the single or multiple nutrient deficiencies so that appropriate and timely treatment can be provided.

When the RDN does not have the skills to conduct an independent nutrition-focused physical exam, physical assessment data from other health care professionals may be used. However, physical assessment findings from another clinician's examination may not adequately document changes in body composition or vitamin/mineral deficiencies. It is therefore important for RDNs to master physical examination skills so they can collect and evaluate data about the patient's nutrition history that are relevant to decisions about the treatment plan.

OVERVIEW OF THE CLINICIAN'S RESPONSIBILITIES

Remember that with privilege comes responsibility. Although it is important to obtain the information that will enhance and complete the nutrition care plan, it is equally important to not subject the patient to unnecessary procedures or discomfort. Table 5.1 summarizes some fundamental obligations of the clinician who performs the physical assessment.

Table 5.1   Responsibilities of Performing Physical Assessment

- Practice universal precautions:
  - Wash hands and clean equipment thoroughly between patient encounters.
  - Wear protective clothing whenever indicated.

(continued)

Table 5.1 Responsibilities of Performing Physical Assessment (continued)

- Respect the patient's privacy and comfort:
  - Inform the patient why the examination is being performed and by whom.
  - Make the patient as comfortable as possible.
  - Allow the patient to empty his or her bladder before examining the abdomen.
  - Keep the patient's body covered except for the area being examined.
- Communicate abnormal findings to the nurse or physician.

AREAS OF FOCUS FOR THE EXAMINATION

Like other health professionals, RDNs should methodically follow a head-to-toe approach when conducting a physical examination. The exam by the RDN focuses on areas that are most influenced by nutrition (see Table 5.2).

Table 5.2 Outline for Performing a Physical Examination

General survey
- Body habitus: Height, weight, BMI[a]
- Level of consciousness
- Gross/fine motor skills
- Contractures
- Amputations
- Vital signs (blood pressure, pulse, respiration, temperature)

Skin, nails, and hair
- Color/uniformity, thickness, moisture, texture, and turgor of skin
- Color and shape of nails
- Color, quantity, and distribution of hair

Head
- Shape
- Symmetry

(continued)

Table 5.2 Outline for Performing a Physical Examination
(continued)

Eyes
- Vision
- Muscle
- Eyelid margin
- Color

Nose
- Shape
- Size
- Nares

Mouth
- Lips
- Teeth
- Gums
- Tongue

Neck and chest
- Symmetry
- Trachea
- Ribs
- Clavicles
- Sternum
- Heart and lung sounds

Abdomen
- Contour/symmetry
- Bowel sounds

Musculoskeletal system
- Size/symmetry
- Muscle tone
- Characteristics
- Strength

[a]See Chapter 4 for more information on assessment of height, weight, and body mass index (BMI).

PHYSICAL EXAMINATION TECHNIQUES

The primary tools required for the examination are gloves and a stethoscope. The primary examination techniques utilized by the RDN include the following:

- **Inspection**: gathering data via observation (Table 5.3)
- **Palpation**: gathering data via touch (for example, touch a patient's arm to determine muscle rigidity or fluid retention) (Table 5.4)
- **Auscultation**: gathering data via listening, such as auscultation of the bowel, heart, or lungs (Tables 5.5–5.7)
- **Percussion**, the act of striking one object against another to produce vibration and sound waves, is not required to perform nutrition-focused physical exam. However, it is important to interpret clinical findings reported in the medical record (Table 5.8).

Figure 5.1 illustrates the four quadrants of the abdomen with anatomical landmarks. Techniques for examining vital signs are described later in this chapter.

Table 5.3   Inspection Techniques

Technique
- Use sight, sense of smell, and hearing to observe textures, sizes, colors, shapes, odors, and sounds

Types of information obtained
- Body composition
- Body habitus: obesity/cachexia
- Fluid status
- Mental status/level of consciousness
- Skin integrity
- Wound healing
- Feeding devices
- Jaundice
- Ascites

Table 5.4   Palpation Technique

Technique
- Use palms and fingertip pads of hands. Use sense of touch. Feel vibrations and pulsations.
  ○ Palpate extremities to assess fluid status and muscle/fat depots.
  ○ Palpate the abdomen in all four quadrants to assess contour and symmetry.
  ○ Use light palpation to assess pulse (jugular, radial, pedal).
  ○ Use deep palpation to assess body structures.
  ○ Palpate tender areas last. Avoid deep palpation of tender areas.

Examples of information obtained
- Areas of tenderness
- Muscle rigidity and distention
- Fluid retention or pitting edema
- Abdominal masses and girth
- Skin integrity and moisture
- Body temperature
- Guarding or rebound tenderness with palpation may indicate peritonitis, perforation, etc

Table 5.5   Auscultation of Bowel Technique

Technique
- Use stethoscope to listen for 3–5 min in the right lower quadrant (RLQ), which is the location of the ileocecal valve.
- If nothing is heard, listen for 1–2 min in the other 3 quadrants.
- Be patient. It could take 10 min to listen effectively to all 4 quadrants.

Examples of information obtained
- *Normal bowel sounds:* Gurgling, high-pitched sounds, heard every 5–15 sec
- Hypoactive bowel sounds:
  ○ Quieter than normal sounds, heard every 15–20 sec
  ○ May indicate paralytic ileus or peritonitis
- Hyperactive bowel sounds:
  ○ Continuous, high-pitched, tinkling sounds
  ○ May indicate diarrhea or intestinal obstruction
- *Absence of sounds:* No sounds after listening for 5 min in RLQ and 2 min in the other 3 quadrants.

(continued)

Table 5.5 Auscultation of Bowel Technique (continued)

Comments
- Absence of bowel sounds is not always a contraindication to enteral feeding.
- Bowel sounds signify the passage of air and fluid. Peristalsis may still occur in the absence of bowel sounds.
- Presence of bowel sounds does not guarantee successful feeding.

Table 5.6 Auscultation of Heart Technique

Technique
- Listen for normal "lub-dub" at the 5 precordial landmarks (noted where sounds can best be heard):
  - Aortic area
  - Pulmonary area
  - Midsternal edge
  - Lower-sterna edge
  - Apex

Examples of information obtained
- Rhythm.
- Murmurs.
- Pericardial friction rub.

Table 5.7 Auscultation of Lungs Technique

Technique
- Listen for abnormal breath sounds.

Examples of information obtained
- Continuous "musical" sounds: wheezing, rhoncus, pleural friction rub
- Discontinuous "brief" sounds (crackles)

Table 5.8 Percussion Technique

Technique
- Use fingertip pads.
- Assess sounds to identify organ border, position, and shape.

Examples of information obtained
- *Abdomen*:
  ○ Tympany suggests obstruction.
  ○ Dullness suggests ascites.
- *Lungs*: Dullness suggests fluid/tissue in place of air.

Comment
- This technique requires practice and acute listening skills.

Figure 5.1 The abdominal quadrants

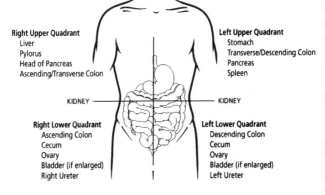

Right Upper Quadrant
Liver
Pylorus
Head of Pancreas
Ascending/Transverse Colon

Left Upper Quadrant
Stomach
Transverse/Descending Colon
Pancreas
Spleen

KIDNEY — — KIDNEY

Right Lower Quadrant
Ascending Colon
Cecum
Ovary
Bladder (if enlarged)
Right Ureter

Left Lower Quadrant
Descending Colon
Cecum
Ovary
Bladder (if enlarged)
Left Ureter

INTERPRETING PHYSICAL EXAMINATION FINDINGS

When interpreting physical examination findings, it is important to note that an isolated nutrient deficiency is rarely identified from this sort of data alone. Signs and symptoms of a deficiency occur after prolonged diet inadequacy. Findings should be correlated with diet history and medical condition (see Chapter 3). Always consider possible nonnutritional causes that could explain the findings.

The following sections provide more detailed information about interpreting data from specific parts of the exam.

GENERAL SYSTEM EXAM INTERPRETATION

Signs of Normal Health

The following general system findings indicate normal health:

- Body weight in normal range for height.
- Body mass index (BMI) in normal range (18.5–24.9)
- Vital signs in normal ranges
- Neurological and psychological stability:
  - Mental orientation to person, place, and time; appropriate responses to questions/environmental stimuli
  - Normal reflexes and sensations
  - Gross and fine motor skills required to complete tasks/activities of daily living

See Chapter 4 for additional information on assessment of body weight and BMI.

Assessment of Vital Signs

Vital signs measure the body's basic functions and are important in medical diagnosis and treatment. For the RDN, assessment of vital signs can provide additional clinical data to help clarify a specific nutrition diagnosis or can further describe an individual's overall clinical picture. Tables 5.9–5.12 review techniques for measuring vital signs and clinical interpretation of the findings (1,8,9).

Table 5.9   Blood Pressure Assessment

Technique
- Allow patient to rest at least 5 min before measuring blood pressure.
- If findings are abnormal, recheck later during the examination to verify.

Clinical interpretation
- Normal: <130 mmHg systolic; <85 mmHg diastolic
- Hypertension: >140 mmHg/90 mmHg (may indicate need for diet therapy)
- Orthostatic hypotension: rapid drop of 25 mmHg when changing from supine to sitting or standing position (associated with hypovolemia)
- If findings are abnormal, assess patient for use of dietary or herbal supplements that can affect blood pressure (eg, yohimbe bark, ma huang/ephedra).

Table 5.10   Radial Pulse Assessment

Technique
- Count pulsations for 15 sec and multiply by 4.
- If pulse is irregular, count for 60 sec.

Clinical interpretation
- Normal: 60–100 pulses/min
- Bradycardia: <60 pulses/min (may be associated with athletes and starvation)
- Tachycardia: >100 pulses/min (may be associated with hypovolemia and caffeine)

Table 5.11   Respiration Assessment

Technique
- Count number of respirations while holding pulse so patient is unaware of monitoring.

Clinical interpretation
- Normal: 14–20 breaths/min
- Labored breathing, chronic obstructive pulmonary disease, or respiratory distress can increase energy expenditure.
- Humidified air reduces insensible fluid loss.

Table 5.12   Temperature Assessment

Technique
- Patient should avoid hot/cold beverages for 10–15 min before measurement.

Clinical interpretation
- Diurnal variation: 35.8°–37.3°C (96.4°–99.1°F)
- Febrile: associated with increased energy expenditure
- Hypothermia or hyperthermia may indicate presence of inflammatory response.

NEUROLOGIC EXAM INTERPRETATION

Table 5.13 lists neurological clinical findings that may indicate nutritional deficiencies (10).

Table 5.13   Selected Neurologic Examination Findings

Clinical Findings	Potential Etiologies
Dementia	• Niacin deficiency • Vitamin B-12 deficiency • Increased calcium • Disease or age related • Medications • Aluminum toxicity

(continued)

Table 5.13   Selected Neurologic Examination Findings
(continued)

Clinical Findings	Potential Etiologies
Confabulation, disorientation	• Thiamin deficiency (Korsakoff's psychosis)
Foot and wrist drop	• Thiamin deficiency
Peripheral neuropathy with weakness and paresthesia; ataxia and decreased tendon reflexes, fine tactile vibrator and position sense	• Thiamin deficiency • Pyridoxine deficiency • Vitamin B-12 deficiency
Tetany	• Calcium deficiency • Magnesium deficiency • Vitamin D deficiency

Source: Data are from reference 10.

SKIN, NAILS, AND HAIR EXAM INTERPRETATION

Skin

When examining skin, signs of normal health are:

• Uniform color
• Smoothness
• A healthy appearance

Table 5.14 lists clinical findings from a skin examination, along with potential nutrition-related etiologies and nonnutrition-related etiologies (10). The online tool Skin Condition Finder (www.skinsight.com/skinCondition Finder.htm) is one resource that includes images of skin disorders; the photos on this site can be sorted by age group, gender, and body part (14).

Table 5.14 Selected Skin Examination Findings

Clinical Findings	Potential Etiologies
Petechiae, especially perifollicular	• Vitamin C deficiency • Abnormal blood clotting • Severe fever • Insect (flea) bite
Ecchymoses	• Vitamin C deficiency • Vitamin K deficiency
Purpura	• Vitamin C deficiency • Vitamin K deficiency • Excessive vitamin E • Warfarin use • Injury • Thrombocytopenia
Follicular hyperkeratosis	• Vitamin A deficiency • Vitamin C deficiency
Spider angioma	• Vitamin B deficiency
Pigmentation; desquamation of sun-exposed areas	• Niacin deficiency
Cellophane appearance	• Protein deficiency • Aging process
Yellow pigmentation of palms of hands with normal white sclera	• Excess beta carotene
Body edema; round, swollen face (moon face)	• Protein deficiency • Thiamin deficiency • Medications, especially steroids
Poor wound healing; decubitus ulcers	• Protein deficiency • Vitamin C deficiency • Zinc deficiency • Kwashiorkor • Poor skin care • Diabetes • Steroid use

(continued)

Table 5.14   Selected Skin Examination Findings (continued)

Clinical Findings	Potential Etiologies
Pallor (may be accompanied by fatigue)	• Iron deficiency • Anemia • Blood loss
Atopic dermatitis	• Niacin deficiency • Zinc deficiency • Food allergy • Contact allergy
Dry, unresilient skin	• Dehydration

Source: Data are from reference 10.

Nails

Uniform, rounded, and smooth nails are an indication of normal health. Table 5.15 lists clinical findings from examination of nails, along with potential nutrition-related etiologies and nonnutrition-related etiologies (10).

Table 5.15   Selected Nail Examination Findings

Clinical Findings	Potential Etiologies
Transverse ridging	• Protein deficiency
Koilonychia	• Iron deficiency • Considered normal if seen on toenails only

Source: Data are from reference 10.

Hair

In an examination of a patient's hair, the following indicate normal health:

- Shiny, firm, not easily plucked hair
- Normal-appearing or thick hair
- Normal-appearing hair shaft and emergence from skin

Table 5.16 lists clinical findings from an examination of hair, along with potential nutrition-related etiologies and nonnutrition-related etiologies (10).

Table 5.16   Selected Hair Examination Findings

Clinical Findings	Potential Etiologies
Flag sign, easily plucked with no pain	• Protein deficiency • Seen in kwashiorkor and occasionally marasmus • Overprocessing hair, as in excess bleaching
Sparse	• Protein deficiency • Biotin deficiency • Zinc deficiency • Alopecia from aging, chemotherapy, or radiation to the head • Endocrine disorders
Corkscrew hair; unemerged, coiled hairs	• Vitamin C deficiency

Source: Data are from reference 10.

HEAD EXAM INTERPRETATION

In the examination of the head, assessment of the shape should take into account variations according to race/ethnicity, gender, and age. The features should normally be symmetric to slightly asymmetric. See Table 5.17 for clinical findings from the examination of the head, along with potential nutrition-related etiologies and nonnutrition-related etiologies (10).

Table 5.17   Selected Head Examination Findings

Clinical Findings	Potential Etiologies
Scaling, nasolabial seborrhea	• Vitamin A deficiency • Vitamin A excess • Zinc deficiency • Riboflavin deficiency • Essential fatty acids deficiency • Pyridoxine deficiency • Nasal congestion
Facial nerve weakness/paralysis affecting swallowing or chewing	• Various illnesses and injuries

Source: Data are from reference 10.

EYE EXAM INTERPRETATION

Figure 5.2 shows the anatomy of the eye.

Figure 5.2   Anatomy of the eye

Reprinted from National Cancer Institute (NCI) Visuals Online.
https://visualsonline.cancer.gov/details.cfm?imageid=1767.

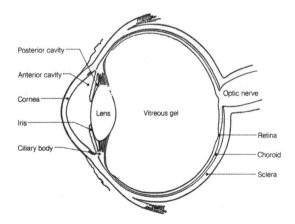

In an eye examination, the following indicate normal health:

- Bright, clear, shiny, smooth cornea
- Pink and moist membranes
- Clear and unapparent conjunctiva
- White sclera
- Normal eye movement to follow objects
- Superior eyelid covering a portion of the iris when open
- Vision 20/20 with or without corrective lenses

Table 5.18 lists clinical findings from an eye examination, along with potential nutrition-related etiologies and nonnutrition-related etiologies (10).

Table 5.18   Selected Eye Examination Findings

Clinical Findings	Potential Etiologies
Pale conjunctiva	• Iron deficiency • Nonnutritional anemia
Night blindness	• Vitamin A deficiency • Heredity • Eye diseases
Bitot's spots	• Vitamin A deficiency
Xerosis	• Vitamin A deficiency
Redness, fissuring in corners of eyes	• Riboflavin deficiency • Pyridoxine deficiency
Ophthalmoplegia	• Thiamin deficiency • Phosphorus deficiency • Brain lesion
Sunken/dry appearance of orbital area	• Dehydration

Source: Data are from reference 10.

NOSE EXAM INTERPRETATION

In the examination of the nose, indicators of normal health include:

- Oval, symmetrically positioned, and pink/glistening mucosa
- Normal sense of smell
- Unobstructed nasal passages (obstructions that interfere with breathing may affect oral intake)

Table 5.19 lists clinical findings from the examination of the nose, along with potential nutrition-related etiologies and nonnutrition-related etiologies.

Table 5.19   Selected Nose Examination Findings

Clinical Findings	Potential Etiologies
Nasogastric suction: • Clear, yellow, green drainage—gastric or small bowel secretions • Brown drainage—possible bowel obstruction • Coffee ground or dark—possible GI bleed	• Gastrointestinal dysfunction
Hyposmia	• Zinc deficiency
Feeding device	• Gastrointestinal dysfunction

Source: Data are from reference 10.

MOUTH EXAM INTERPRETATION

Figure 5.3 shows the anatomy of the mouth.

Figure 5.3   Mouth and facial anatomy

Reprinted from National Cancer Institute (NCI) Visuals Online.
https://visualsonline.cancer.gov/details.cfm?imageid=1780.

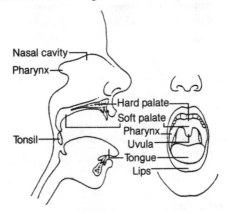

In an oral examination, the following are indicators of
normal health:

- Lips smooth, with distinct borders, and without sores
- Tongue dull red, moist, glistening, and without
  swelling
- Normal surface
- Normal taste
- Normal gums (slightly stippled and pink)
- Normal, firmly anchored teeth

Table 5.20 lists clinical findings from the examination of
the mouth, along with potential nutrition-related etiologies and nonnutrition-related etiologies (10).

Table 5.20   Selected Mouth Examination Findings

Clinical Findings	Potential Etiologies
Cheilosis, angular stomatitis	• Riboflavin deficiency • Pyridoxine deficiency • Niacin deficiency • Excessive salivation due to ill-fitting dentures • Dehydration • Dry skin (winter)
Atrophic lingual papillae	• Riboflavin deficiency • Niacin deficiency • Folate deficiency • Vitamin B-12 deficiency • Protein deficiency • Iron deficiency
Hypoguesia	• Zinc deficiency • Medications such as antineoplastic agents or sulfonylureas • Nasal congestion
Mottled tooth enamel	• Excess fluoride
Eroded enamel	• Bulimia
Cavities, missing teeth	• Poor dental hygiene
Retracted gums	• Periodontal disease
Swollen, bleeding gums; retracted gums with teeth	• Vitamin C deficiency • Poor oral hygiene • Pregnancy
Lip pallor	• Anemia
Parotid enlargement	• Protein deficiency • Bulimia • Disease of the parotid • Excess vitamin A

Source: Data are from reference 10.

NECK AND CHEST EXAM INTERPRETATION

Figure 5.4 shows the anatomy of the chest.

Figure 5.4   Anatomy of the chest

Reprinted from National Cancer Institute (NCI) Visuals Online: https://visualsonline.cancer.gov/details.cfm?imageid=1774.

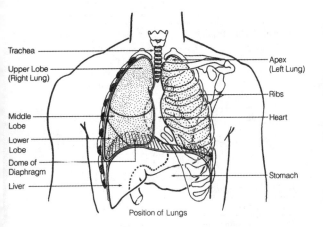

Position of Lungs

Indicators of normal health in the neck and chest examination include the following:

- Bilateral symmetry of the sternocleidomastoid and trapezius muscles
- Trachea in midline position
- Prominent ribs with clavicles noticeable superiorly
- Chest somewhat asymmetric
- Flat sternum
- Normal heart and lung sounds (see Tables 5.6 and 5.7, earlier in this chapter, for more information on auscultation of heart and lungs)

Physical examination findings with possible nutritional implications include:

- Jugular vein distention (may indicate fluid overload)
- Feeding or vascular access device
- Tracheostomy
- "Pigeon" chest (horizontal depression along the lower border of chest—may indicate vitamin D deficiency)
- Costochondral beading/rachitic rosary (may indicate vitamin D deficiency)
- Abnormal heart or lung sounds

ABDOMINAL EXAM INTERPRETATION

In the examination of the abdomen, the following are signs of normal health:

- A flat, rounded, or scaphoid abdomen
- Normal bowel sounds (see Table 5.5, earlier in this chapter, for more information on bowel sounds)
- Absence of a feeding device

Table 5.21 lists clinical findings in the abdomen that may indicate a nutrition-related problem (10).

Table 5.21　Selected Abdomen Examination Findings

Clinical Findings	Potential Etiologies
Umbilicus displaced upward, downward, or laterally	• Gastrointestinal dysfunction
Abdominal pain	• Gastrointestinal dysfunction
Scar/wound/ostomy	• Gastrointestinal dysfunction

(continued)

Table 5.21   Selected Abdomen Examination Findings
               (continued)

Clinical Findings	Potential Etiologies
High-pitched, tinkling bowel sounds	• Gastrointestinal dysfunction
Decreased or absent bowel sounds	• Gastrointestinal dysfunction
Feeding device	• Gastrointestinal dysfunction
Hepatomegaly	• Protein deficiency • Bulimia • Liver disease • Excess vitamin A

Source: Data are from reference 10.

MUSCULOSKELETAL EXAM INTERPRETATION

Physical signs of normal musculoskeletal health include:

- Approximately symmetric bilateral muscle size with firm muscle tone
- Bilaterally symmetric strength with full resistance to opposition
- Minimal fat wasting
- No edema

Table 5.22 lists clinical findings in the musculoskeletal examination that may indicate a nutrition-related problem (10–11).

Table 5.22   Selected Musculoskeletal Examination Findings

Clinical Findings	Potential Etiologies
Inability to produce expected strength	• Muscle wasting • Protein-energy deficiency
Head: depression or concave temple region	• Possible loss of temporalis muscle • Protein-energy deficiency
Head: darken under-eye circles, sunken region under the eye with loose skin	• Possible depletion of orbital fat pads • Protein-energy deficiency
Chest/back/upper extremity: prominent clavicle and/or scapula, visible/protruding acromion process, squared appearance to shoulder/deltoid	• Possible loss of pectoralis major, trapezius, supraspinatus, infraspinatus or deltoid muscle • Protein-energy deficiency
Chest/back/upper extremity: prominent ribs and/or iliac crest	• Possible depletion of subcutaneous fat surrounding the thoracic and abdominal region • Protein-energy deficiency
Lower extremity: wasted appearance to calf/quadriceps, prominent patella/medial epicondyle (femur)/lateral epicondyle (femur) medial condyle (tibia)/lateral condyle (tibia)	• Possible loss of quadriceps, hamstring, gastrocnemius, or soleus muscle • Protein-energy deficiency
Rickets or osteomalacia	• Calcium deficiency

Source: Data are from reference 10 and 11.

HYDRATION STATUS

Along with laboratory data (see Chapter 6), physical examination findings help determine a patient's hydration status. Refer to Tables 5.23 and 5.24 for parameters for evaluating dehydration and overhydration (1,8,9,14).

Table 5.23   Dehydration (Fluid Deficit)

Clinical Findings	Potential Etiologies
Vital sign aberrations:	*Inadequate fluid intake:*
• Decreased blood pressure	• IV fluids
• Decreased cardiac output	• Oral fluid intake
• Decreased central venous pressure	• Tube feeding flushes
• Decreased pulmonary artery	*Excessive losses:*
wedge pressure	• Diaphoresis
• Increased heart rate	• Diarrhea/emesis
• Increased temperature	• NG/fistula/drains/ostomy
• Increased systemic vascular	• Dialysis, hemofiltration
resistance	• Persistent fevers
Physical findings:	• Wounds, burns,
• Input <output	paracentesis
• Decreased weight	• Hemorrhage
• Sunken, dry eyes	• Polyuria
• Dark colored urine, oliguria	• Medications
• Dry mucous membranes	• Anabolism
• Sticky saliva	
• Poor skin turgor	
• Cool, pale, clammy skin	
• Jugular vein flattened (< 3 cm	
when flat or lying down)	
Mental effects:	
• Dizziness	
• Confusion	

Source: Data are from references 1, 8, 9, and 14.

Table 5.24   Overhydration (Fluid Excess)

Clinical Findings	Potential Etiologies
Vital-sign aberrations:	*Excessive fluid intake:*
• Increased blood pressure	• Surgical procedures
• Increased cardiac output	• IV fluids
• Increased central venous pressure	*Interstitial fluid retention:*
	• Hypoalbuminemia
• Increased pulmonary artery wedge pressure	*Disease processes:*
Physical findings:	• Renal failure
• Input > output	• Liver failure, ascites
• Increased weight	• Congestive heart failure
• Puffy, swollen eyes	• Syndrome of inappropriate antidiuretic hormone (SIADH)
• Light colored urine	
• Moist skin	• Severe hypertension
• Edema (peripheral and sacral)	
• Anasarca	
• Shortness of breath, dyspnea, lung crackles	
• Jugular vein distention (>3 cm when sitting up)	

Source: Data are from references 1, 8, 9, and 14.

REFERENCES

1. Bickley LS. *Bates' Guide to Physical Examination and History Taking.* 10th ed. Philadelphia, PA: Wolters Kluwer Health/Lippincott Williams & Wilkins; 2009.

2. Seidel H, Ball JW, Dains JE, Benedict GW. *Mosby's Guide to Physical Examination.* 7th ed. St. Louis, MO: Mosby/Elsevier; 2011.

3. Cashman M, Sloan S. Nutrition and nail disease. *Clin Dermatol.* 2010;28(4):420–425.

4. Goldberg L, Lenzy Y. Nutrition and hair. *Clin Dermatol.* 2010;28(4):412–419.

5. Jen M, Yan A. Syndromes associated with nutritional deficiency and excess. *Clin Dermatol.* 2010;28(6):669–685.

6. Moccia LDR. Abdominal examination: A guide for dietitians. *Support Line.* 2011;33(2):16.

7. Pogatshnik C, Hamilton C. Nutrition-focused physical examination: Skin, nails, hair, eyes and oral cavity. *Support Line.* 2011;33(2):7.

8. Elkin MK, Perry AG, Potter PA, eds. *Nursing Interventions and Clinical Skills.* St. Louis, MO: Mosby; 1996.

9. Murphy LM, Bickford V. Physical assessment of cardio-pulmonary system: Nutrition implications. *Support Line.* 1997;19(2):8–11.

10. Morrison SG. Clinical Nutrition physical examination. *Support Line.* 1997;19(2):16–18.

11. White J, Guenter P, Jensen, G. Consensus statement of the Academy of Nutrition and Dietetics/American Society for Parenteral and Enteral Nutrition: Characteristics recommended for the identification and documentation of adult malnutrition (under-nutrition). *J Acad Nutr Diet.* 2012;112:730–738.

12. Fischer M, JeVenn A, Hipskind P. Evaluation of muscle and fat loss as diagnostic criteria of malnutrition. *Nutr Clin Pract* 2015;30:239–248.

13. Saltzman E, Karl JP. Nutrient deficiencies after gastric bypass surgery. *Annu Rev Nutr.* 2013;33:183–203.

14. Pesce-Hammond K, Wessel J. Nutrition assessment and decision making. In: Merritt R, ed. *The A.S.P.E.N. Nutrition Support Practice Manual.* 2nd ed. Silver Springs, MD: American Society for Parenteral and Enteral Nutrition; 2006:3–37.

14. Skin Condition Finder. www.skinsight.com/skinCondition Finder.htm. Accessed April 15, 2015.

Chapter 6

Biochemical Tests, Medical Data, and Procedures

Cheryl W. Thompson, PhD, RD, CNSC

INTRODUCTION

Accurate interpretation of laboratory data requires knowledge of the appropriate test to order as well as the nutritional and nonnutritional factors that alter blood chemistries. A complete diet history, including supplement usage and physical signs/symptoms, can provide important supportive information. See Chapter 3 for more information on food and nutrition-related history.

Nonnutritional factors, such as disease processes, treatments, procedures, medications, and hydration status, can profoundly alter blood and urine chemistries and must be considered. Blood levels can also be carefully controlled by homeostatic mechanisms and may not reflect tissue stores. Ideally, any nutrition-related laboratory test should evaluate tissue stores or nutrient function.

Keep in mind:

- A review of serial laboratory data is recommended. The direction and speed of change can be more important than a static value.
- Assay methods vary greatly. Use reference values established by your laboratory.

- An improvement in nutrition parameters does not always confer clinical benefit. Improved clinical outcome remains the ultimate goal.
- Treat the patient, not the laboratory value. Abnormal laboratory reports that are unexpected or inconsistent with the clinical picture should be repeated before treatment.

HEPATIC TRANSPORT PROTEIN ASSESSMENT

There is no laboratory test that is both sensitive to and specific for protein-calorie malnutrition. Evaluation of serum albumin, transferrin, and prealbumin is no longer recommended as a component of the nutrition assessment.

Acute-Phase Response

The acute-phase response is a systemic response to acute or chronic inflammation associated with conditions such as infection, trauma, surgery, and cancer. Mediators, such as cytokines, that are released in the response, cause the liver to reprioritize the synthesis of proteins to those most critical for host defense and adaptive capabilities. Increased protein degradation and transcapillary losses also occur. Therefore, the serum concentrations of some proteins will increase while others decrease.

An acute-phase response increases the C-reactive protein concentration, along with other positive acute-phase reactants, such as ceruloplasmin, ferritin, and others, while simultaneously decreasing albumin, transferrin, prealbumin, and retinol-binding protein. Regardless of nutrition support, these protein levels will not return to normal until the inflammatory stress subsides.

Elevated temperature and/or white blood cell count can be general indications of an inflammatory response. In addition, an increased C-reactive protein concentration or erythrocyte sedimentation rate (ESR) can be helpful in quantifying the intensity of an acute-phase response. However, the clinical examination would provide the same information. Therefore, routine monitoring of C-reactive protein is not warranted and additional costs must be considered, especially when multiple measurements are necessary to evaluate a trend (1).

Albumin

In unstressed starvation, normal albumin levels are preserved because of decreased catabolism and increased mobilization of the body's extravascular stores (where approximately 60% of the body's albumin pool is found) (2). Albumin is neither sensitive to, nor specific for, acute protein malnutrition or the response to nutrition therapy.

During a critical illness, factors that alter serum albumin include the following:

- The acute-phase response
- Hydration (intravascular volume) status
- Disease state
- Clinical condition
- Leakage of albumin from intravascular to extravascular spaces

Blood loss and perioperative fluid resuscitation will also contribute to rapid decreases in postoperative albumin levels. One consequence of hypoalbuminemia is a reduction in colloid osmotic pressure, with a corresponding shift of intravascular fluid into extravascular spaces, which may be evident as edema or ascites (2).

While albumin has some use as a prognostic indicator of morbidity, mortality, and severity of illness, it has little to no correlation with nutritional status (see Table 6.1). Hypoalbuminemia has been associated with increased hospital length of stay, morbidity (eg, postoperative complications, infection, organ dysfunction), and mortality in numerous studies (3,4). However, other noninvasive prognostic indicators such as sepsis scoring and the APACHE II score probably provide more information and have greater reliability.

Table 6.1   Factors That Decrease or Increase Albumin

Interpretation of laboratory values
- Normal: 3.5–5 g/dL
- Mild depletion: 3–3.4 g/dL
- Moderate depletion: 2.4–2.9 g/dL
- Severe depletion: <2.4 g/dL
- Half-life: approximately 14–20 days

Factors that *decrease* albumin
- Acute-phase response[a]
- Severe liver failure
- Redistribution: intravascular volume overload, third spacing, pregnancy, minor decrease with recumbency
- Increased losses: nephrotic syndrome, burns, protein-losing enteropathies, exudates
- Severe zinc deficiency

Factors that *increase* albumin
- Intravascular volume depletion
- Intravenous albumin or plasminate, blood transfusions (temporary rise)
- Anabolic steroids, possibly glucocorticoids

[a]Acute-phase response occurs with inflammation associated with conditions such as infection, injury, surgery, and cancer.

Transferrin

Compared to albumin, transferrin has a smaller and primarily intravascular body pool and shorter half-life. The primary function of transferrin is to bind and transport iron. Therefore, synthesis of transferrin is inversely correlated with the body's iron stores.

An elevated transferrin concentration often indicates early iron deficiency. It is also the last laboratory value to return to normal when iron deficiency is corrected. In addition to iron status, an awareness of the acute-phase response must be considered because transferrin levels will decrease during acute illness (see Table 6.2).

Table 6.2   Factors That Decrease or Increase Transferrin

Interpretation of laboratory values
- Normal: 200–400 mg/dL
- Mild depletion: 150–200 mg/dL
- Moderate depletion: 100–149 mg/dL
- Severe depletion: <100 mg/dL
- Half-life: approximately 8–10 days

Factors that *decrease* transferrin
- Acute-phase response
- Chronic or end-stage liver disease
- Uremia
- Protein-losing states (some nephrotic syndromes, burns)
- Intravascular volume overload
- High-dose antibiotic therapy (such as amino-glycosides, tetracycline, and some cephalosporins)
- Iron overload
- Severe zinc deficiency

Factors that *increase* transferrin
- Iron deficiency, chronic blood loss
- Pregnancy (markedly increases in 3rd trimester)
- Intravascular volume depletion
- Acute hepatitis
- Oral contraceptives, estrogen

Although direct measurement of serum transferrin is more accurate, several equations are available to calculate transferrin from the total iron-binding capacity (TIBC). Depending on which equation is used, the calculated transferrin concentration can vary greatly. Verify with the laboratory which equation is most closely correlated with its assay methods.

Prealbumin (Transthyretin, Thyroxin-Binding Prealbumin)

Prealbumin is a carrier protein for thyroxin (thyroid hormone) and, combined with retinol-binding protein, transports vitamin A. Compared with albumin or transferrin, it has a shorter half-life, a smaller plasma pool, is influenced less by intravascular fluid volume, and is not affected as early or as significantly with liver disease.

Cost and lack of specificity and sensitivity limit the usefulness of prealbumin as a screening or assessment tool. Prealbumin is known to decline rapidly with an acute-phase response and therefore is subject to similar limitations in interpretation as albumin and transferrin. In stable renal failure (such as chronic hemodialysis) or with the use of corticosteroids, prealbumin will be elevated and should not be used to diagnose nutrition problems. See Table 6.3 for more information on interpretation of prealbumin.

Table 6.3   Factors That Decrease or Increase Prealbumin

Interpretation of laboratory values
- Normal: 16–40 mg/dL
- Mild depletion: 10–15 mg/L
- Moderate depletion: 5–9 mg/dL
- Severe depletion: <5 mg/dL
- Half-life: approximately 2–3 days

Factors that *decrease* prealbumin
- Acute-phase response
- End-stage liver disease (hepatitis, cirrhosis)
- Untreated hyperthyroidism
- Nephrotic syndrome
- Severe zinc deficiency

Factors that *increase* prealbumin
- Moderate increase in acute or chronic renal failure
- Anabolic steroids, possibly glucocorticoids

IMMUNE FUNCTION PARAMETERS

Delayed cutaneous hypersensitivity and reduced total lymphocyte count are two tests that have been used to quantify the impaired immune function associated with uncomplicated malnutrition. However, they are no longer used as part of a routine assessment of hospitalized patients because the inflammatory processes and some therapies, such as chemotherapy and steroids, alter the results (5).

BLOOD GLUCOSE ASSESSMENT

Prediabetes, Type 1 Diabetes Mellitus, and Type 2 Diabetes Mellitus

Diabetes mellitus is a state of chronic hyperglycemia resulting from a deficiency of insulin and/or resistance to the action of insulin.

- Individuals with **type 1 diabetes** do not produce appreciable amounts of endogenous insulin and are dependent on exogenous insulin for survival.
- Those with **type 2 diabetes** have either a relative lack of endogenous insulin, impaired insulin receptor function (insulin resistance), or both and can be treated with diet, oral hypoglycemic agents, insulin, or a combination of these three therapies.

Screening and Diagnosis

Although marked hyperglycemia is symptomatic, mild to moderate elevations in blood glucose are often asymptomatic and can go undetected. American Diabetes Association (ADA) and American Association of Clinical Endocrinologists/American College of Endocrinology

(AACE/ACE) recommendations for diabetes testing in asymptomatic adults age are summarized in Table 6.4 (6,7). Table 6.5 explains the use of glucose testing and A1C for the diagnosis of prediabetes and diabetes (6,7). (A1C is described in greater detail later in this chapter.)

Table 6.4   AACE/ACE and ADA Diabetes Screening Criteria for Asymptomatic Adults[a]

Age
- Screening recommended for all asymptomatic adults age ≥45 y with or without additional risk factors

BMI
- ADA: Screening recommended for all asymptomatic adults with BMI ≥25 (≥23 in Asian Americans) if they have additional risk factors
- AACE/ACE: Screening recommended for all asymptomatic adults with BMI ≥25 (at-risk BMI may be lower in some ethnic groups with additional risk factors; waist circumference and other parameters may be used for individuals in these groups)

Additional risk factors
- CVD
- Family history of type 2 diabetes (AACE/ACE) / first-degree relative with diabetes (ADA)
- Sedentary lifestyle (AACE/ACE) / physical inactivity (ADA)
- Member of an at-risk/high-risk racial or ethnic group:
  - African American
  - Asian
  - Hispanic/Latino
  - Native American
  - Pacific Islander
- HDL-C <35 mg/dL (0.9 mmol/L)
- TG >250 mL/dL (2.82 mmol/L)
- HTN (BP >140/90 mmHg or on HTN therapy)
- Acanthosis nigricans

(continued)

**Table 6.4   AACE/ACE and ADA Diabetes Screening Criteria for
Asymptomatic Adults[a]** (continued)

- PCOS
- NAFLD (AACE/ACE)
- Any clinical conditions associated with insulin resistance (ADA)
- History of GDM
- Past delivery of baby weighing >4 kg (9 lb)
- IGT or IFG
- Metabolic syndrome (AACE/ACE)
- A1C ≥5.7% (ADA)
- Antipsychotic therapy for schizophrenia or severe bipolar disease (AACE/ACE)
- Chronic glucocorticoid exposure (AACE/ACE)
- Sleep disorders in the presence of glucose intolerance (A1C >5.7%, IGT, or IFG on previous testing, including OSA, chronic sleep deprivation, and night-shift occupation (AACE/ACE)

Timing and frequency of testing
- AACE/ACE: At-risk individuals whose glucose values are normal should be screened at least every 3 years. Consider annual screening for individuals with ≥2 risk factors.
- ADA: At-risk individuals whose glucose values are normal should be screened at least every 3 years. Consider whether more frequent screening is appropriate for at-risk individuals. Test individuals with prediabetes annually.

Abbreviations: A1C, hemoglobin A1C; AACE/ACE, American Association of Clinical Endocrinologists/American College of Endocrinology; ADA, American Diabetes Association; BMI, body mass index; BP, blood pressure; CVD, cardiovascular disease; GDM, gestational diabetes mellitus; HDL-C, high-density lipoprotein cholesterol; HTN, hypertension; IFG, impaired fasting glucose; IGT, impaired glucose tolerance; NAFLD, nonalcoholic fatty liver disease; OSA, obstructive sleep apnea; PCOS, polycystic ovary syndrome; TG, triglycerides.

[a]Unless otherwise noted, criteria are the same for AACE/ACE and ADA.

Source: Data are from references 6 and 7.

Table 6.5   Interpretation of Glucose Testing and Diagnosis of Prediabetes and Diabetes[a]

FPG[b]

- Normal: < 100 mg/dL
- High-risk for diabetes (prediabetes): 100–125 mg/dL (5.6–6.9 mmol/L)[c,d]
- Diabetes: ≥126 mg/dL (7 mmol/L)

2-hour PG

- Normal: < 140 mg/dL
- High-risk for diabetes (prediabetes): 140–199 mg/dL (7.8–11 mmol/L)[d,e]
- Diabetes: ≥200 mg/dL (11.1 mmol/L)[f]

A1C[g]

- Normal: < 5.5% (AACE/ACE); < 5.7% (ADA)
- High-risk for diabetes (prediabetes): 5.5%–6.4% (AACE/ACE); 5.7%–6.4% (ADA)[d]
- Diabetes: ≥6.5%

Abbreviations: A1C, hemoglobin A1C; AACE/ACE, American Association of Clinical Endocrinologists/American College of Endocrinology; ADA, American Diabetes Association; FPG, fasting plasma glucose; PG, plasma glucose
[a]AACE/ACE recommends confirmation of diabetes diagnosis on a separate day by repeating glucose or A1C testing (glucose criteria are preferred) (11). ADA recommends confirmation of diabetes diagnosis by repeat testing in all cases except those involving unequivocal hyperglycemia (6).
[b]Fasting is defined as no caloric intake for ≥8 hours (6).
[c]FPG 100–125 mg/dL (5.6–6.9 mmol/L) = impaired fasting glucose.
[d]Prediabetes risk is continuous, extending below the lower limit of the range and becoming disproportionately greater at higher ends of the range (6).
[e]2-h PG 140–199 mg/dL (7.8–11 mmol/L) = impaired glucose tolerance.
[f]Random PG ≥200 mg/dL (11.1 mmol/L) plus hyperglycemic symptoms also indicates diabetes.
[g]According to AACE/ACE, A1C should be used only for screening prediabetes. The diagnosis of prediabetes should be confirmed with glucose testing. When A1C is used for diagnosis, follow-up glucose testing should be done, if possible, to help manage diabetes (11).
Source: Data are from references 6 and 7.

Insulin Therapy and Blood Glucose Targets

Early studies of intensive insulin therapy to achieve tight glycemic control (80–110 mg/dL) found reduced morbidity and mortality in diabetic and nondiabetic critically ill surgical patients compared to conventional treatment to maintain glucose between 180 and 200 mg/dL (8,9); with less dramatic results in medical intensive care patients (10). A 2009 meta-analysis concluded that intensive insulin therapy may benefit surgical patients, but no overall mortality benefit was found in a mixed critically ill population (11).

The following guidelines are based on 2015 recommendations of the ADA and AACE/ACE (6,7) as well as the AACE/ADA 2009 consensus statement (12):

- In the hospital setting, blood glucose >140 mg/dL (7.8 mmol/L) is considered hyperglycemia (6).
  - A target for most nonpregnant adult inpatients is 140–180 mg/dL (7.8–10 mmol/L) if it can be achieved safely (7). Initiate insulin therapy starting at a threshold of ≤180 mg/dL (10 mmol/L).
  - For most critically ill patients with persistent hyperglycemia, a goal of 140–180 mg/dL (7.8–10 mmol/L) is appropriate (6).
  - Select patients may benefit from stricter goals (eg, 110–140 mg/dL [6.1–7.8 mmol/L]) as long as significant hypoglycemia can be avoided. (6).
  - Targets <110 mg/dL (6.1 mmol/L) are not recommended (7,12).
- Each hospital should adopt a hypoglycemia management protocol that includes plans to prevent, treat, and document occurrences (6,7). Promptly identify and treat mild-to-moderate hypoglycemia (40–69 mg/dL [2.2–3.8 mmol/L]) to prevent adverse consequences (6).

- Reasonable goals for most noncritically ill patients treated with insulin are premeal blood glucose targets generally <140 g/dL (7.8 mmol/L) with random blood glucose <180 mg/dL (10 mmol/L), if these can be safely achieved (6,7,12). Use professional judgment and ongoing assessment of clinical status to tailor the patient's regimen to maintain glycemic control (7).
- Hospitals should initiate glucose monitoring with bedside point-of-care (POC) testing in all patients with known diabetes and in other patients receiving therapy associated with high risk of hyperglycemia, such as corticosteroids or enteral or parenteral nutrition (7). For patients who are eating, monitoring four to six times per day is typical. Patients who are nil per os or receiving continuous enteral nutrition should have POC testing every four to six hours (7,12). More frequent glucose monitoring is indicated in patients treated with continuous intravenous insulin infusion or after a medication change that could alter glycemic control, such as corticosteroid use, abrupt discontinuation of enteral or parenteral nutrition, or frequent episodes of hypoglycemia (7).
- Point of care glucose meters may be less reliable in conditions of low/high hemoglobin, hypoperfusion or some medications (12). If results are inconsistent with the patient's clinical status, confirm using regular laboratory methods.

In patients with diabetes, chronic hyperglycemia is associated with an increased risk of microvascular (retinopathy, nephropathy, and neuropathy) and macrovascular (coronary heart disease and peripheral vascular and cerebrovascular disease) complications. Intensive glycemic control clearly reduces the onset of microvascular and neurologic complications (13). One long-term trial found that tight glycemic control was associated with a reduced risk of cardiovascular complications in type 1 diabetes (14). Nevertheless, large clinical trials are necessary to clarify the extent to which tight glycemic control can prevent or delay macrovascular complications in type 1 and type 2 diabetes (13).

The AACE/ACE guidelines encourage all patients with diabetes to maintain glycemic control as close to normal as possible without causing clinically significant hypoglycemia. The following general goals of therapy are recommended for most nonpregnant adults (7):

- Fasting glucose < 110 mg/dL
- 2-hour postprandial glucose < 140 mg/dL
- A1C level ≤ 6.5% (A1C is discussed in greater detail later in this chapter)

Screening in Pregnancy and Gestational Diabetes Mellitus

Pregnant women with risk factors for diabetes should be tested for type 2 diabetes at the first prenatal visit (use standard criteria; see Table 6.5) (7).

At 24 to 28 weeks' gestation, the risk of adverse maternal, fetal, and neonatal outcomes increases even within glycemic ranges previously considered normal for pregnancy. Screening criteria for GDM are presented in Table 6.6 (6,7). Additionally, ADA has published a two-step screening method (6).

**Table 6.6   Screening for and Diagnosis of Gestational Diabetes
                  Mellitus**

Testing method
- Screen patient at 24–28 weeks' gestation.
- If patient does not have previous diagnosis of diabetes,
  measure PG via a 75-g OGTT when she is fasting,[a] at 1 hour,
  and at 2 hours.

GDM diagnostic criteria
  ○ FPG: >92 mg/dL (5.1 mmol/L)
  ○ 1-h PG: 180 mg/dL (10 mmol/L)
  ○ 2-h PG: 153 mg/dL (8.5 mmol/L)

Abbreviations: FPG, fasting plasma glucose; GDM, gestational diabetes mellitus; OGTT, oral glucose tolerance test; PG, plasma glucose.
[a]Perform OGTT in the morning, following a fast of ≥8 hours (6).
Source: Data are from references 6 and 7.

Evaluating Blood Glucose Levels

Abnormalities in blood glucose most commonly occur in
type 1 or type 2 diabetes (6,15,16). However, the differential diagnoses include the factors listed in Tables 6.7
and 6.8.

Table 6.7   Potential Causes and Symptoms of Hypoglycemia

Potential causes
- Treatment of diabetes:
  ○ Dose of insulin or oral agent is excessive, inappropriately
    timed, or the wrong type
  ○ Inadequate glucose (missed meal)
  ○ Increased glucose use (exercise)
  ○ Increased insulin sensitivity (effective intensive therapy)
  ○ Decreased endogenous glucose production (alcohol)
  ○ Decreased insulin clearance (renal failure)

                                                         (continued)

Table 6.7   Potential Causes and Symptoms of Hypoglycemia
(continued)

- Medications:
  - Insulin
  - Oral hypoglycemic agents (especially sulfonylureas)
  - Alcohol
  - Pentamidine
- Fasting hypoglycemia:
  - Critical illness (severe hepatic or renal disease, sepsis)
  - Non-β-cell tumors
  - Insulinoma
- Postprandial (reactive) hypoglycemia:
  - Idiopathic
  - Rapid gastric emptying (eg, postgastrectomy)
  - Abrupt discontinuation of PN or other rapid dextrose infusions
- Deficient counterregulatory hormones:[a]
  - Glucagon and/or epinephrine (type 1 DM)
  - Cortisol or growth hormone deficiency (rare)

Potential symptoms

- Sweating
- Tremor
- Anxiety
- Tachycardia
- Hunger
- Weakness
- Dizziness
- Headache
- Confusion that may progress to seizures and loss of consciousness

Abbreviations: PN, parenteral nutrition; DM, diabetes mellitus.
[a]Glucagon, cortisol, catecholamines (epinephrine and norepinephrinc) and growth hormone.

Table 6.8   Potential Causes and Symptoms of Hyperglycemia

Potential causes
- Diabetes mellitus:
  - Type 1 (autoimmune or idiopathic beta-cell destruction)
  - Type 2 (insulin resistance or relative insulin deficiency)
  - Gestational (insulin resistance)
- Impaired exocrine pancreas:
  - Pancreatitis
  - Pancreatectomy
  - Pancreatic cancer
  - Hemochromatosis
  - Cystic fibrosis
  - Rare genetic defects
- Medications:
  - Glucocorticoids
  - Thiazide diuretics[a]
  - Phenytoin
  - Epinephrine
- Excess counterregulatory hormones:[b]
  - Trauma
  - Infection
  - Autonomous endocrine diseases (eg, acromegaly, Cushing syndrome, pheochromocytoma, glucagonoma, hyperthyroidism)
- Excessive dextrose:
  - High-dextrose IV fluid or PN
  - Absorption from high-dextrose dialysate fluid
- Chromium deficiency (very rare)

Potential symptoms
- Polyuria
- Polydipsia
- Polyphagia
- Weight loss
- Fatigue
- Blurred vision
- Impaired wound healing
- Increased susceptibility to infection

Abbreviations: IV, intravenous; PN, parenteral nutrition.
[a]Thiazide diuretics include hydrochlorothiazide, chlorthalidone, indapamide, and metolazone.
[b]Glucagon, cortisol, catecholamines (epinephrine and norepinephrine) and growth hormone.

Monitoring Long-Term Glucose Control: A1C

Glycated hemoglobin (the A1C test or HbA1c) reflects the patient's mean plasma glucose (MPG) level during the preceding two to three months (6). The correlation between A1C and MPG concentrations have been modified based on expanded data (6):

- A1C 6% = MPG 126 mg/dL (7 mmol/L)
- A1C 7% = MPG 154 mg/dL (8.6 mmol/L)
- A1C 8% = MPG 183 mg/dL (10.2 mmol/L)
- A1C 9% = MPG 212 mg/dL (11.8 mmol/L)
- A1C 10% = MPG 240 mg/dL (13.4 mmol/L)
- A1C 11% = MPG 269 mg/dL (14.9 mmol/L)
- A1C 12% = MPG 298 mg/dL (16.5 mmol/L)

The A1C test reflects the amount of glucose bound to hemoglobin over the lifespan of the red blood cells (RBC). Consequently, results are falsely low in diseases that shorten RBC lifespan (eg, sickle cell, hemolytic anemias, and chronic blood loss) and are falsely high after a splenectomy (15).

A1C and Diagnosis of Diabetes

Refer to Table 6.5, earlier in this chapter, for A1C values used in the diagnosis of diabetes (6,7).

Frequency of A1C Testing

A baseline A1C test measurement should be evaluated upon diagnosis of diabetes mellitus. Frequency of monitoring the A1C test will depend on the treatment regimen and judgment of the clinician. It is recommended that the test be given (6):

- At least two times a year for patients who are meeting treatment goals and whose glycemic control is stable
- Every three months for patients whose therapy has changed or who are not meeting glycemic goals

A1C Goals

- A reasonable A1C goal for many nonpregnant adults is <7% (6). AACE/ACE recommends A1C ≤6.5% (7) as a general goal, if it is achievable.
- More stringent goals (eg, <6.5%) are recommended for some patients (eg, those with short duration of diabetes, long life expectancy, and no significant cardiovascular disease) if such goals are feasible without significant hypoglycemia (6).
- Less stringent goals (eg, <8%) may be recommended for patients with a history of severe hypoglycemia, limited life expectancy, advanced microvascular or macrovascular complications, or extensive comorbid conditions. Less stringent goals may also be advisable for patients with long-standing diabetes who cannot achieve the general goal of A1C <7% even when following a regimen of self-management, glucose monitoring, and glucose-lowering medications (6,7).
- Compared with goals for adults, A1C goals for children and adolescents can be higher (<7.5%) because of the risk for impairment of cognitive function by frequent hypoglycemic events; however, a lower goal (<7%) may be reasonable for some pediatric patients if it can be achieved without excessive hypoglycemia (6).

Diabetic Ketoacidosis and Hyperosmolar, Hyperglycemic State

Insulin deficiency, increased counterregulatory hormones, and volume depletion can result in diabetic ketoacidosis (DKA) or hyperosmolar, hyperglycemic state (HHS), occurring most frequently in type 1 and type 2 diabetes, respectively (17). See Table 6.9 (17).

Table 6.9   Laboratory Abnormalities Often Seen with Diabetic Ketoacidosis and Hyperosmolar, Hyperglycemic State

Laboratory Abnormalities	Diabetic Ketoacidosis (Mild to Severe)	Hyperosmolar Hyperglycemic State
Hyperglycemia	Plasma glucose >250 mg/dL	Plasma glucose >600 mg/dL
Ketosis:[a] ketones in urine and/or blood	Positive	Small
Metabolic acidosis	Arterial pH <7–7.3 Serum bicarbonate <10–18 mEq/L Anion gap >10–12	pH >7.3 Serum bicarbonate >15 mEq/L Anion gap variable
Electrolyte shifts	Despite a total-body deficit, serum potassium is initially normal to elevated, then drops rapidly with correction of the acidosis, insulin therapy, and volume expansion	Normal serum potassium
Serum osmolality	Variable	>320 mOsm per kg water

[a]Nitroprusside reaction method. Ketosis is also seen in alcoholism, starvation, very low–carbohydrate diets, and up to 30% of first-morning urine samples during pregnancy.
Source: Data are from reference 17.

ELECTROLYTE ASSESSMENT

Sodium

Hyponatremia and hypernatremia are disorders of sodium (Na) concentration in the serum, not of total-body sodium. Serum sodium concentrations correlate poorly with the need for sodium repletion and are typically more reflective of total-body water than sodium balance.

Evaluation of abnormal serum sodium concentrations requires a simultaneous examination of volume status to determine the cause and appropriate therapy.

Hyponatremia

Hyponatremia is defined as serum sodium <135 mEq/L. Hyponatremia can be present with decreased, normal, or increased total-body water and/or sodium. True sodium depletion (decreased total-body sodium) is uncommon. However, it can occur as a result of the replacement of gastrointestinal (GI) or renal losses with free water or other hypotonic fluids (eg, D_5W [5% dextrose in water], .25 NS [normal saline], or .5 NS). For more information on this topic, refer to references 15, 16, and 18–22.

Symptoms of hyponatremia are uncommon unless serum sodium declines rapidly or falls below ~120 to 125 mEq/L, at which point nausea, vomiting, headache, lethargy, and mental-status changes (eg, confusion or psychosis) can occur. In cases of severe hyponatremia (~ <115 mEq/L), convulsions, seizures, coma, and even death may occur. The correction of hyponatremia should proceed at a gradual rate because aggressive treatment can precipitate neurologic sequelae (central pontine myelinolysis).

An important step in diagnostic evaluation of hyponatremia is to measure or calculate serum osmolality.

[eq]Calculated Serum Osmolality = [2 × Serum Na (mEq/L)] + [Serum Glucose (mg/dL)/18] + [Serum BUN (mg/dL)/2.8]

When hyponatremia is associated with decreased serum osmolality (<280 mOsm/kg H_2O), it is essential to simultaneously evaluate the patient's volume status (ie, extracellular fluid volume [ECF]). As indicated in Table 6.10 (19,21,22), this will help determine the etiology and appropriate treatment (see also the Hydration Status sections of this chapter and Chapter 5: Nutrition-Focused Physical Assessment). Table 6.11 (19,21,22) outlines the etiologies and treatment when hyponatremia is associated with an increased or normal serum osmolality, which are less common manifestations of hyponatremia.

Table 6.10   Evaluation of Hyponatremia When Serum Osmolality Is Low (< 280 mOsm/kg H_2O)

ECF finding: volume depletion (hypovolemic hypotonic hyponatremia)
Definition:
  • Total-body water deficit with larger total-body sodium deficit
Signs and symptoms:
  • Tachycardia, low blood pressure, decreased skin turgor
  • Urine Na^+ <20 mEq/L usually indicates extrarenal losses
  • Urine Na^+ >20 mEq/L usually indicates renal losses
Possible causes:
  • Extrarenal losses:
    ° GI tract: diarrhea (especially secretory), vomiting, gastric suction, fistula
    ° Skin: burns, excessive sweating
    ° Third spacing: ascites, bowel obstruction, peritonitis, pancreatitis
    ° Lungs: bronchorrhea
  • Renal losses:
    ° Diuretics
    ° Renal disease: renal tubular acidosis, salt-wasting nephropathy
    ° Osmotic diuresis: ketones, glucose, urea
    ° Primary adrenal insufficiency
Treatment:
  • Treat underlying cause.
  • Volume expansion; replete with isotonic fluids (eg, NS or lactated Ringer's)
  • Replace ongoing losses with fluids containing a similar composition.

(continued)

Table 6.10   Evaluation of Hyponatremia When Serum Osmolality Is Low (< 280 mOsm/kg H_2O) (continued)

ECF finding: euvolemic or modest ECF volume excess (isovolemic hypotonic hyponatremia)

Definition:
- Normal to moderately increased total-body water ± total-body sodium

Signs and symptoms:
- Normal pulse, blood pressure and skin turgor; no edema
- Urine Na^+ usually >20 mEq/L

Possible causes:
- SIADH
- Glucocorticoid deficiency
- Hypothyroidism
- Polydipsia
- Reset osmostat syndrome (cachexia, malnutrition)
- Iatrogenic (eg, renal failure with provision of hypotonic fluid exceeding excretory capacity)
- Potassium depletion

Treatment:
- Treat underlying cause
- Water restriction

ECF finding: volume expansion (hypervolemic hypotonic hyponatremia)

Definition:
- Excess total-body sodium with larger excess of total-body water

Signs and symptoms:
- Edema
- Urine Na^+ <20 mEq/L usually indicates edema-forming states
- Urine Na^+ >20 mEq/L usually indicates renal failure

Possible causes:
- Edema-forming states: congestive heart failure, cirrhosis, nephrotic syndrome
- Acute or chronic renal failure

Treatment:
- Treat underlying cause
- Sodium and water restriction

Abbreviations: ECF, extracellular fluid; GI, gastrointestinal; Na+, sodium; NS, normal saline; SIADH, syndrome of inappropriate antidiuretic hormone.
Source: Data are from references 19, 21, and 22.

Table 6.11   Evaluation of Hyponatremia When Serum Osmolality Is Normal (280–295 mOsm/kg H20) or High (> 295 mOsm/kg H20)

Normal serum osmolality (iso-osmolar hyponatremia)

Possible causes:

- Infusion of isotonic, sodium-free solutions (eg, during transurethral resection of the prostate or bladder)
- Pseudohyponatremia[b]

Treatment:

- Treat underlying cause.

High serum osmolality (hyperosmolar hyponatremia)

Possible causes:

- Hyperglycemia[a]
- Infusion of hypertonic, sodium-free solutions (eg, mannitol)
- Toxins

Treatment:

- Treat underlying cause.

---

[a]Serum sodium is falsely decreased by approximately 1.6 mEq/L for each 100 mg/dL rise in glucose. The adjustment in serum sodium should be calculated in hyperglycemic conditions.

[b]Pseudohyponatremia is an artificially low sodium concentration that can occur (with hyperlipidemia or hyperproteinemia) if using the flame photometric laboratory techniques and does not warrant treatment to correct hyponatremia.

Source: Data are from references 19, 21, and 22.

Hypernatremia

Hypernatremia is defined as serum sodium >145 mEq/L. For more information on this topic, refer to references 15, 16, and 18–22.

Hypernatremia is much less common than hyponatremia but is associated with a high morbidity and mortality. Sodium is the main cation in ECF and, along with accompanying anions, is the primary determinant of serum osmolality.

Hypernatremia essentially never occurs in a patient with a normal thirst mechanism and access to water. The elderly are at risk of dehydration because of declining renal sodium conservation and diminished thirst perception.

The onset of symptoms will depend on both the rate and degree of increased serum sodium.

- Early signs include thirst and dry mucous membranes.
- Neurologic signs, such as drowsiness, lethargy, disorientation, and confusion, are observed as water progressively shifts from intracellular fluid (ICF) spaces into the hyperosmolar ECF.
- Severe hypernatremia can result in respiratory paralysis, coma, and ultimately death.

Serum osmolality is not useful to evaluate the etiology of hypernatremia because it is always elevated in hypernatremic states. However, it can be useful to monitor the severity and progress of correction.

As hypernatremia reflects a derangement of the relative amounts of sodium and water, an evaluation of hypernatremia must be done in conjunction with an assessment of volume status to identify the etiology and appropriate treatment strategy. Most commonly, hypernatremia is associated with a water deficit (dehydration) and is rarely due to a gain in total-body sodium. An exception, however, is in patients with traumatic brain injury in whom a hyperosmolar state is desired.

An estimation of free-water deficit can be calculated using serum sodium levels:

$$\text{Free-Water Deficit (liters)} = \{1 - [140/\text{Serum Na (mEq)}]\} \times [0.6 \times \text{Actual Body Weight (kg)}]$$

Refer to Table 6.12 (21,22) for information regarding the evaluation of ECF and hypernatremia. See also the Hydration Status sections of this chapter and Chapter 5.

Table 6.12   Hypernatremia and Evaluation of Extracellular Fluid Volume

---

ECF finding: volume depletion (hypovolemic hypernatremia)
Definition:
- Total-body sodium deficit with larger total-body water deficit
Urine Na$^+$:
- <20 mEq/L indicates extrarenal losses
- >20 mEq/L indicates renal losses
Possible causes:
- Extrarenal losses:
  ◦ GI tract: severe diarrhea (especially osmotic), vomiting, fistula losses
  ◦ Skin: excessive sweating, burns
  ◦ Lungs: bronchorrhea, hyperventilation
- Renal losses:
  ◦ Diuresis: diuretics, osmotic diuresis (glucosuria, diuretic phase of acute tubular necrosis)
  ◦ Partial urinary tract obstruction
  ◦ Renal dysplasia
Treatment:
- Volume expansion:
  ◦ Initially use isotonic fluids (eg, NS, lactated Ringer's)
  ◦ After hemodynamic stability and good urine output, change to hypotonic saline.

ECF finding: euvolemia or modest ECF volume loss (isovolemic hypernatremia)
Definition:
- Total-body water loss with normal total-body sodium
Urine Na$^+$:
- Variable
Possible causes:
- Extrarenal losses:
  ◦ Skin losses: especially if replacement is NS
  ◦ Lung losses: hyperventilation
  ◦ Water deprivation: inadequate access to water, hypodypsia
- Renal losses:
  ◦ Diabetes insipidus (central or nephrogenic)
Treatment:
- Treat underlying cause
- Water replacement

(continued)

Table 6.12   Hypernatremia and Evaluation of Extracellular Fluid Volume (continued)

ECF finding: volume expansion[a] (hypervolemic hypernatremia)

Definition:
- Total-body sodium excess greater than total-body water excess (uncommon)

Urine Na+:
- >20 mEq/L

Possible causes:
- Iatrogenic sodium administration: inappropriate use of NaCl, NaHCO$_3$, hypertonic dialysis, high-sodium medications (salt tablets, sodium-salt antibiotics), or—rarely—excess dietary sodium
- Mineralocorticoid excess: hyperaldosteronism, Cushing's disease, congenital adrenal hyperplasia

Treatment:
- Decrease sodium in intravenous fluids, PN, and medications.
- Remove sodium with diuretics (or dialysis, if in renal failure).
- Water replacement

Abbreviations: ECF, extracellular fluid; GI, gastrointestinal; NS, normal saline; NaCl, sodium chloride; NaHCO$_3$, sodium bicarbonate; PN, parenteral nutrition.

[a]In hypervolemic hypernatremia, overt evidence of ECF volume expansion may not be evident on physical examination.

Source: Data are from references 21 and 22.

Potassium

Potassium (K) is the major intracellular fluid (ICF) cation, with less than 2% of total-body stores in ECF. Normal serum potassium is 3.5–5.0 mEq/L. For more information on this topic, refer to references 15, 16, 18, 20, and 22.

Hypokalemia

Serum levels of potassium do not correlate well with body stores. However, in the absence of acid-base disturbances or transcellular shifts, a low serum potassium level may provide a rough estimation of the depleted body stores:

- A decline in serum potassium from 4.0 to 3.0 mEq/L may correlate with an estimated deficit of 200–400 mEq.
- A serum potassium level <3.0 mEq/L may require >600 mEq to replete body potassium stores.

Frequent monitoring is required to assess the response during repletion. With refractory hypokalemia, serum magnesium should also be monitored, as potassium repletion is impaired in magnesium-deficient states. See Table 6.13 for more information on hypokalemia.

Table 6.13   Potential Etiologies and Signs/Symptoms of Hypokalemia

Potential etiologies
- Renal losses:
  - Osmotic diuresis
  - Hypomagnesemia
  - Hyperaldosteronism, Cushing's syndrome, or Bartter's syndrome
  - Licorice excess
- GI losses:
  - Diarrhea
  - Intestinal or biliary fistula
  - Ureterosigmoidostomy
  - Villous adenoma
  - Prolonged vomiting or gastric suction
- Medications:
  - Loop[a] or thiazide[b] diuretics
  - Amphotericin B
  - Cisplatin
  - Insulin
  - Beta$_2$ adrenergic agonists[c]
  - Foscarnet
  - High-dose glucocorticoids or penicillins

(continued)

**Table 6.13   Potential Etiologies and Signs/Symptoms of
Hypokalemia** (continued)

- Shift into cells:
  - Alkalosis
  - Anabolism
  - Refeeding syndrome
  - Correction of hyperglycemia or DKA
- Inadequate intake (seldom the sole cause):
  - Anorexia nervosa
  - Malnutrition
  - Alcoholism
  - IV hydration without potassium

Signs and symptoms
- Potassium ~ <3.0 mEq/L:
  - Muscle weakness
  - Myalgias
  - Constipation
  - Ileus
  - Decreased deep-tendon reflexes
- EKG changes:
  - Flat or inverted T wave
  - Increased U wave
  - Depressed ST segment
  - Arrhythmias

Abbreviations: GI, gastrointestinal; DKA, diabetic ketoacidosis; IV, intravenous; EKG, electrocardiogram.
[a]Loop diuretics include furosemide, bumetanide, ethacrynic acid, torsemide.
[b]Thiazide diuretics include hydrochlorothiazide.
[c]Beta$_2$ adrenergic agonists include isoproterenol, epinephrine, terbutaline.

Hyperkalemia

Chronic hyperkalemia is usually due to impaired renal excretion. A spurious elevation in serum potassium is possible if the blood sample is hemolyzed during phlebotomy or if it contains very high platelets (thrombocytosis) or white blood cells (leukocytosis).

Serum potassium can also be falsely elevated if the blood is drawn from a vein or an inadequately flushed IV line into which potassium is being infused (eg, PN). If the blood sample is contaminated with PN, the glucose will typically also be elevated. A repeat blood sample should be obtained. Serum potassium is increased by approximately 0.6 mEq/L for each 0.1-drop in pH, or decreased 0.6 with each 0.1-increase in pH. Correction of an acid-base disturbance will adjust the serum potassium level. See Table 6.14 for more information on hyperkalemia.

Table 6.14   Potential Etiologies and Signs/Symptoms of Hyperkalemia

Potential etiologies
- Decreased renal excretion:
  ◦ Acute oliguric renal failure
  ◦ Chronic renal failure
  ◦ Hypoaldosteronism
  ◦ Type IV renal tubular acidosis
- Medications:
  ◦ Potassium sparing diuretics[a]
  ◦ Beta blockers[b]
  ◦ ACE inhibitors[c]
  ◦ Cyclosporine
  ◦ Heparin
  ◦ Digitalis toxicity
  ◦ Trimethoprim
  ◦ Tacrolimus
  ◦ Pentamidine
  ◦ NSAIDs
- Shift out of cells:
  ◦ Acidosis
  ◦ Massive cellular destruction (tissue necrosis, rhabdomyolysis, GI hemorrhage, hemolysis, hemolytic anemia)

(continued)

Table 6.14   **Potential Etiologies and Signs/Symptoms of Hyperkalemia** (continued)

Signs and symptoms
- Muscle weakness, paresthesias, decreased deep-tendon reflexes, flaccid paralysis
- Potassium ~>7.0 mEq/L is potentially life-threatening, with EKG changes: peaked T waves; prolonged PR interval, wide QRS, small or absent P waves, ventricular arrhythmias. Finally, QRS degenerates into a sine wave and cardiac arrest.

Abbreviations: ACE, angiotensin-converting enzyme; NSAIDs, nonsteroidal anti-inflammatory drugs; GI, gastrointestinal; EKG, electrocardiogram.
[a]Potassium-sparing diuretics include amiloride, triamterene, spironolactone.
[b]Beta blockers include propranolol, metoprolol, and atenolol; they rarely cause hyperkalemia alone but contribute to elevations with other conditions.
[c]ACE inhibitors include captopril, enalapril, quinapril, and ramipril.

Calcium

Normal serum calcium (Ca) is 9–10.5 mg/dL. Normal ionized calcium is 4.5–5.6 mg/dL. For more information on this topic, refer to references 15, 16, 18, 20, 21, and 23.

Less than 1% of the body's calcium is present in ECF. Normal serum calcium levels are primarily maintained by hormonal regulation (parathyroid hormone, vitamin D, and calcitonin). Large skeletal reserves help to compensate for inadequate calcium intake or reduced GI absorption (seen with a diet high in phosphorus, oxalate, or phytate). Total serum calcium reflects the ionized calcium, plus calcium bound to protein (primarily albumin) and anions.

Hypocalcemia

The equations to adjust serum calcium for hypoalbuminemia are not reliable for use in acute care because of poor sensitivity and a high rate of false negatives (23). Ionized calcium is a more accurate reflection of the physiologically active calcium level and should be evaluated before initiating calcium repletion, especially in patients with hypoalbuminemia. Furthermore, serum magnesium and phosphorus levels should also be measured and, if low, treated in patients with hypocalcemia. See Table 6.15 for more information on hypocalcemia.

Table 6.15   Potential Etiologies and Signs/Symptoms of Hypocalcemia

Potential etiologies
- Hypoalbuminemia[a]
- Hypoparathyroidism
- Hypomagnesemia
- Renal failure, renal tubular acidosis
- Vitamin D deficiency or impaired metabolism
- Medications:
  - Foscarnet
  - Loop diuretics[b]
  - Anticonvulsants[c]
  - Cisplatin
  - Plicamycin
  - Gentamicin
  - Corticosteroids
  - Calcitonin
  - Colchicine
  - Denosumab
- Hyperphosphatemia
- Acute pancreatitis
- Hungry bone syndrome[d]
- Citrated blood products

Signs and symptoms
- Often asymptomatic; symptoms reflect degree and acuteness of decline in serum.
- Paresthesias of fingers/toes/mouth, muscle cramps, nonspecific psychiatric changes
- Severe (ionized calcium ~<2 mg/dL or 0.5 mmol/L):
  - Positive Chvostek's[e] or Trousseau's sign[f]
  - Tetany, muscle spasms, hyperactive reflexes
  - EKG changes: prolonged QT and ST intervals
  - Convulsions, seizures, refractory hypotension, arrhythmias, bradycardia, cardiac arrest

(continued)

Table 6.15   **Potential Etiologies and Signs/Symptoms of Hypocalcemia** (continued)

- Chronic:
  - Dry/scaly skin
  - Brittle nails
  - Coarse hair
  - Cataracts

[a]The total serum calcium level will be decreased by hypoalbuminemia; however, the ionized calcium will be unchanged. Obtain an ionized calcium level or calculate the corrected calcium:

$$\text{Corrected Ca} = \text{Total Serum Ca (mg/dL)} + \{0.8 \times [4 - \text{Serum Albumin (g/dL)}]\}$$

[b]Loop diuretics include furosemide, bumetanide, ethacrynic acid.
[c]Anticonvulsants include phenobarbital, phenytoin, carbamazepine, primidone.
[d]Hungry bone syndrome occurs in some patients after a parathyroidectomy and is characterized by rapid/excessive osteogenesis that can result in hypocalcemia.
[e]Chvostek's sign: A twitch of the facial muscles upon tapping the facial nerve in front of the ear.
[f]Trousseau's sign: A hand spasm observed when the blood pressure cuff is inflated to above systolic blood pressure for up to 3 minutes.

Hypercalcemia

Typically, hypercalcemia occurs when excessive calcium from the intestine and/or bone enters the ECF and exceeds the renal excretory capacity (see Table 6.16).

Table 6.16   **Potential Etiologies and Signs/Symptoms of Hypercalcemia**

Potential etiologies
- Hyperparathyroidism
- Some malignancies (with or without metastasis to the bone), especially breast, lung, or kidney; multiple myeloma, leukemia, or lymphoma

(continued)

Table 6.16 **Potential Etiologies and Signs/Symptoms of
Hypercalcemia** (continued)

- Medications:
  ○ Thiazide diuretics[a]
  ○ Lithium
  ○ Vitamin A toxicity
- Immobilization
- Hyperthyroidism
- Less common causes: Excess 1,25-dihydroxyvitamin D,
  tuberculosis, sarcoidosis, milk-alkali syndrome, after renal
  transplantation, diuretic phase of acute renal failure

Signs and symptoms
- Mild:
  ○ Often asymptomatic; typically nonspecific
- Symptomatic (total calcium ~> 11.5 mg/dL):
  ○ Nausea, vomiting
  ○ Anorexia
  ○ Polydipsia, polyuria, dehydration
  ○ Muscle weakness, fatigability, hyporeflexia
  ○ Constipation
  ○ Mental changes, confusion, depression
  ○ EKG changes: shortened QT interval, bradyarrhythmias ~> 18
    mg/dL may cause shock, renal failure, coma, death
- Chronic:
  ○ With increased phosphorus, hypercalcemia can cause soft-
    tissue deposits,[b] hypertension

Abbreviation: EKG, electrocardiogram.
[a]Thiazide diuretics include hydrochlorothiazide.
[b]The calcium-phosphorus product—ie,
   [serum Ca (mg/dL)] × [serum P (mg/dL)]—should not be > 70 mg/dL.

Phosphorus

Normal serum phosphorus (P) is 3–4.5 mg/dL. For more
information on this topic, refer to references 15, 16, 18,
20, and 21.

Phosphorus is the primary intracellular anion. The
serum phosphorus level is a poor reflection of body stores
because < 1% is present in ECF, and the bones serve as a

reservoir that can buffer changes in serum or intracellular phosphorus.

Hypophosphatemia

Despite the limitations of the serum phosphorus level in the assessment of body stores, it can serve as a rough guide for recommendations for empiric replacement. Oral or enteral supplementation is the preferred route when the GI tract is functional. However, intravenous replacement therapy is usually warranted in profound hypophosphatemia (<1 mg/dL) if the patient is symptomatic or when oral replacement therapy is limited by GI side effects. Response to supplementation is unpredictable and should be monitored closely. Delaying or holding nutrition support intervention until repletion has occurred warrants consideration. See Table 6.17 for more information.

Table 6.17   Potential Etiologies and Signs/Symptoms of Hypophosphatemia

Potential etiologies
- Impaired absorption:
  - Malabsorption
  - Diarrhea
  - Vitamin D deficiency or impaired metabolism
- Medications:
  - Phosphate-binding antacids[a]
  - Sucralfate
  - Steroids (anabolic and glucocorticoid)
  - Insulin
  - Epinephrine
- Alcoholism
- Intracellular shifts:
  - Alkalosis (especially respiratory)
  - Cellular uptake (anabolism, some neoplasms)
  - Burn (especially recovery)
  - Sepsis

(continued)

Table 6.17   Potential Etiologies and Signs/Symptoms of Hypophosphatemia (continued)

- Refeeding syndrome
- Increased losses:
  - Hyperparathyroidism
  - Renal tubular defects (Fanconi syndrome)
  - DKA (the recovery phase)
  - Hypomagnesemia
  - Diuretic phase of ATN (briefly) or after renal transplantation
- Inadequate intake:
  - PN or dextrose-based IVF without adequate phosphorus

Signs and symptoms
- Mild:
  - Usually asymptomatic
- Severe (Phosphorus < 1–1.5 mg/dL):
  - Anorexia
  - Confusion, irritability
  - Muscle weakness, paresthesias, decreased diaphragmatic contractility, ataxia, seizure
  - RBC dysfunction
  - Thrombocytopenia
  - Hemolysis
  - Rhabdomyolysis
  - Coma
  - Respiratory failure/arrest

Abbreviations: DKA, diabetic ketoacidosis; ATN, acute tubular necrosis; PN, parenteral nutrition; IVF, intravenous fluid; RBC, red blood cell.
[a]Phosphate-binding antacids include those that are aluminum based (aluminum hydroxide) and those that are calcium based (calcium acetate, carbonate, or gluconate).

Hyperphosphatemia

Hyperphosphatemia is most commonly due to impaired renal excretion. Serum phosphorus can be artificially elevated by hemolysis of the blood sample. Thrombocytosis and multiple myeloma can also cause spurious elevations. See Table 6.18 for more information.

Table 6.18   Potential Etiologies and Signs/Symptoms of Hyperphosphatemia

Potential etiologies
- Decreased renal excretion:
  - Acute or chronic renal failure
  - Hypoparathyroidism
  - Acromegaly
- Increased cellular release:
  - Tumor lysis syndrome
  - Tissue necrosis
  - Rhabdomyolysis
- Increased exogenous phosphorus load or absorption:
  - Phosphorus-containing laxatives or enemas
  - Vitamin D excess
- Acidosis (shift into ECF)

Signs and symptoms
- Usually asymptomatic
- Hypocalcemia
- Chronic:
  - If calcium-phosphorus product remains > 70 mg/dL, soft-tissue deposits or joint calcification may occur

Abbreviation: ECF, extracellular fluid.

Magnesium

Normal serum magnesium (Mg) is 1.3–2.1 mEq/L. Serum levels may not accurately reflect body stores because only about 1% of magnesium is present in ECF. For more information on this topic, refer to references 15, 16, 18, 20, and 21.

Hypomagnesemia

Hypomagnesemia is usually due to inadequate intake in conjunction with increased renal losses or impaired GI absorption. Magnesium depletion is commonly seen in critically ill patients, people with alcoholism, and in patients with diabetes who have osmotic diuresis.

Hypocalcemia and hypokalemia are frequently associated with hypomagnesemia and are refractory to repletion until the magnesium deficit is corrected. Clinical manifestations of hypomagnesemia are similar to hypocalcemia and can be exacerbated if both are present.

Oral magnesium replacement can result in diarrhea. Intravenous or intramuscular repletion is recommended for severe and/or symptomatic cases. See Table 6.19 for more information on hypomagnesemia.

Table 6.19   Potential Etiologies and Signs/Symptoms of Hypomagnesemia

Potential etiologies
- Decreased absorption:
  - Prolonged diarrhea
  - Intestinal or biliary fistula
  - Intestinal resection or bypass
  - Steatorrhea
  - Ulcerative colitis
  - To a lesser extent, upper GI fluid losses (prolonged gastric suction, excessive vomiting)
- Renal losses:
  - Osmotic diuresis
  - DM/glucosuria
  - Correction of DKA
  - Renal disease with magnesium wasting
  - Hypophosphatemia
  - Hypercalcemia
  - Hyperthyroidism
  - Hyperaldosteronism
  - Diuretic phase of acute tubular necrosis
  - Renal tubular acidosis
  - Inherited renal tubular defects
- Alcoholism
- Inadequate intake: Malnutrition

(continued)

Table 6.19   Potential Etiologies[a] and Signs/Symptoms of Hypomagnesemia (continued)

- Medications:
  - Diuretics[a]
  - Amphotericin B
  - Aminoglycosides[b]
  - Cisplatin
  - Cyclosporine
  - Pentamidine
  - Foscarnet
  - Tacrolimus
- Intracellular shift: Acute pancreatitis
- Refeeding syndrome

Signs and symptoms
- Magnesium ~ <0.5–1 mEq/L:
  - Muscle weakness, muscle tremors progressing to seizures, tetany
  - Anorexia
  - Nausea
  - Mental status changes (confusion, depression, psychosis)
  - Hypocalcemia with positive Chvostek's sign[c] or, less frequently, positive Trousseau's sign[d]
  - EKG changes: Flat or inverted T wave (a sign of either hypomagnesemia or hypokalemia), increased PR and QT interval, ventricular arrhythmias

Abbreviations: GI, gastrointestinal; DM, diabetes mellitus; DKA, diabetic ketoacidosis; EKG, electrocardiogram.
[a]Mild hypomagnesemia can occur with loop or thiazide diuretics.
[b]Aminoglycoside antibiotics include gentamicin and tobramycin.
[c]Chvostek's sign: A twitch of the facial muscles upon tapping the facial nerve in front of the ear.
[d]Trousseau's sign: A hand spasm observed when the blood pressure cuff is inflated to above systolic blood pressure for up to three minutes.

Hypermagnesemia

Normal kidneys can excrete excess magnesium efficiently; therefore, chronic hypermagnesemia is usually associated with renal failure. Symptomatic hypermagnesemia is fairly uncommon. See Table 6.20 for more information.

Table 6.20   Potential Etiologies[a] and Signs/Symptoms of Hypermagnesemia

Potential etiologies
- Acute or chronic renal failure
- The following seldom cause significant/chronic hypermagnesemia unless renal function is also impaired:
  - Medications: magnesium-rich cathartics and antacids,[b] administration of magnesium to suppress premature labor
  - Rhabdomyolysis
  - Adrenal insufficiency (Addison's disease)
  - Hypothyroidism
  - Dehydration

Signs and symptoms
- Diminished deep-tendon reflexes
- EKG changes: prolonged PR interval; also peaked T wave, wide QRS complex (can be either hypermagnesemia or hyperkalemia), arrhythmias
- Mental confusion
- Respiratory depression, respiratory muscle paralysis, peripheral vasodilation resulting in profound hypotension
- Magnesium ~> 12–15 mEq/L can cause cardiac arrest

Abbreviation: EKG, electrocardiogram.

[a]Note that laboratory error may lead to incorrect serum magnesium results. Artificial increases are seen with hemolysis or decreases with hypoalbuminemia.

[b]Magnesium-rich cathartics include magnesium citrate and milk of magnesia. Magnesium-containing antacids include Maalox and Mylanta.

ACID-BASE ASSESSMENT

pH is a measure of acidity/alkalinity based on the number of hydrogen ions (H^+) present:

- **Acids** by definition are H^+ donors, such as hydrochloric acid
- **Bases** are H^+ acceptors, including bicarbonate, acetate, citrate, lactate, and gluconate.

The arterial pH is maintained within a narrow physiologic range (7.35–7.45) by the combined action of the lungs, via control of the partial pressure of carbon dioxide in the blood (PCO_2), and of the kidneys via control of bicarbonate and acid excretion and the production of buffers. Some nonrenal buffer systems also exist. For more on this topic, refer to references 15, 18, 19, 21, and 24.

Types of Acid-Base Disorders

Acid-base disorders can be metabolic or respiratory:

- Metabolic acid-base disorders manifest as changes in serum chloride and bicarbonate (HCO_3).
- Respiratory acid-base disorders are characterized by abnormalities in PCO_2.

The body attempts to compensate for a primary *metabolic* acid-base disorder with "secondary" or "compensatory" *respiratory* changes. The lungs usually respond within minutes to compensate by adjusting minute ventilation (ie, respiratory rate × tidal volume), in order to retain or release carbon dioxide. Large amounts of acid can be removed when hydrogen ions (H^+) are buffered by bicarbonate and converted to water and CO_2, which is expired by the lungs.

Conversely, hypoventilation can help to conserve acid. A primary *respiratory* acid-base disorder typically elicits a compensatory *renal* response.

The kidneys retain or excrete acid (H^+) and/or base equivalents to maintain serum pH. The occurrence of metabolic compensation takes several hours to days, even in the healthy kidney. Buffers present in body fluids, such as bicarbonate, hemoglobin, proteins, ammonium, and phosphates, can act immediately to help maintain a normal pH.

Evaluation and Treatment of Acid-Base Disorders

To evaluate an acid-base disturbance, the pH and PCO_2 are obtained from an arterial blood gas (ABG) sample, along with measurement of serum CO_2 (which consists primarily of HCO_3), sodium, and chloride. Serial measurements are collected and interpreted in conjunction with the patient's clinical status and, if mechanically ventilated, the ventilatory parameters.

Remember to treat the primary disorder—not the compensatory mechanism. If the expected compensation does not occur, it may indicate a second primary disorder (mixed acid-base disorder). However, mixed acid-base disorders are beyond the scope of this pocket guide.

Some metabolic acid-base imbalances may respond to adjustments in acetate and/or chloride content of parenteral nutrition and other IV fluids. Respiratory imbalances will not.

However, if a primary respiratory acidosis cannot be corrected by supporting lung function, metabolic compensation may be augmented by adjusting the acetate load of the PN. The composition of enteral feeding will not alter acid-base disturbances. However, if medium-chain triglyceride (MCT) oil is provided in excess of oxidative capacity, increased ketone bodies are produced, which may worsen acidosis.

Overfeeding results in excess CO_2 production. If this exacerbates an acute respiratory acidosis, calories should be limited to maintenance requirements.

See Tables 6.21 through 6.24 for additional information on acid-base disorders.

Table 6.21   Expected Compensation, Causes, and Treatment of Metabolic Acidosis

Uncompensated acidosis
- Low pH (<7.35)
- Low HCO_3^- (<21 mEq/L)
- Normal PCO_2 (35–45 mmHg)

Compensated acidosis
- Near normal pH
- Low HCO_3^-
- Low PCO_2
- Respiratory compensation occurs by increasing respiratory rate and/or depth (hyperventilation). PCO_2 should fall approximately 1.3 mm Hg for each 1-mEq/L drop in HCO_3^-.

Principal causes
- Increased anion gap acidosis[a] (normochloremic metabolic acidosis):
  ○ Ketoacidosis (diabetic, alcoholic, starvation)
  ○ Lactic acidosis (hypoperfusion, shock, severe liver failure, thiamin deficiency)
  ○ Acute or chronic renal failure
  ○ Toxic acid ingestion (ethylene glycol, methanol, paraldehyde, salicylate overdose)
- Normal anion gap acidosis[a] (hyperchloremic metabolic acidosis)
- GI HCO_3^- loss:
  ○ Diarrhea
  ○ Small bowel/biliary/pancreatic drainage or fistula
  ○ Ureterosigmoidostomy
- Renal HCO_3^- loss, impaired reabsorption, or impaired H^+ excretion:
  ○ Renal tubular acidosis
  ○ Interstitial nephritis
  ○ Hypoaldosteronism
  ○ Early renal insufficiency
  ○ Obstructive nephropathy
- Iatrogenic:
  ○ Carbonic anhydrase inhibitors (acetazolamide)
  ○ Excess chloride from NS, PN, or acidifying agents (ammonium chloride, hydrochloric acid)

(continued)

Table 6.21   Expected Compensation, Causes, and Treatment of Metabolic Acidosis (continued)

Treatment
- Correct underlying defect.
- Supplementation with alkali (eg, sodium bicarbonate[b]) or bicarbonate precursors (eg, sodium citrate) may be appropriate in some cases.
- In PN, increase acetate if significant and/or chronic HCO_3^- losses.[b] Decrease chloride if acidosis is due to excess.
- Hyperkalemia usually resolves with correction of acidosis.

Abbreviations: HCO_3^-, bicarbonate; PCO_2, partial pressure of carbon dioxide; GI, gastrointestinal; NS, normal saline; PN, parenteral nutrition; Na, sodium; Cl, chloride.

[a]The anion gap is based on the concept that there is a normal difference between the primary measured cation (Na^+) and anions (Cl^-, HCO_3^-). This difference or "gap" helps to determine the etiology of metabolic acidosis because it is increased when other unmeasured anions are present. Anion gap = $(Na^+) - (Cl^- + HCO_3^-)$. A normal anion gap is 8–12 mEq/L, although it can vary significantly with different laboratories.

[b]Bicarbonate is unstable in PN and is not added because of the risk of precipitation. Acetate and/or lactate are used as bicarbonate precursors that are converted to bicarbonate in the liver.

Table 6.22   Expected Compensation, Causes, and Treatment of Metabolic Alkalosis

Uncompensated alkalosis
- High pH (>7.45)
- High HCO_3^- (>24 mEq/L)
- Normal PCO_2 (35–45 mmHg)

Compensated alkalosis
- Near normal pH
- High HCO_3^-
- High PCO_2
- Respiration is depressed (hypoventilation) as a compensatory response by the lungs. PCO_2 typically rises about 0.7 mm Hg for each 1-mEq/L increase in HCO_3^-.

(continued)

Table 6.22 Expected Compensation, Causes, and Treatment of Metabolic Alkalosis (continued)

Principal causes
- Chloride-responsive alkalosis:[a]
  - GI loss of chloride and/or acid (gastric drainage, vomiting, laxative abuse, colonic villous adenoma)
  - Diuretics; volume contraction
  - Correction of chronic hypercapnia
- Chloride-unresponsive alkalosis:[a]
  - Excess mineralocorticoid—Cushing syndrome, primary hyperaldosteronism, glucocorticoids, glycyrrhizic acid/licorice, Bartter syndrome
- Other:
  - Excess alkali intake: Citrate (Shol's solution, massive blood transfusions, regional citrate anticoagulation during continuous renal replacement therapy); HCO_3^- (NaHCO$_3$, Ringer's lactate, acetate), excessive antacids, PN with excess acetate
  - Intracellular H^+ shift: Severe potassium depletion

Treatment
- Correct underlying defect. Replete deficit of chloride, potassium, magnesium, and/or volume. If possible, stop gastric suction, diuretics, and/or excess bicarbonate.
- In PN, increased chloride can be appropriate in the chloride-responsive categories listed above or acetate can be decreased when excess alkali is the cause.
- Monitor for hypokalemia from renal tubule losses plus a shift from ECF to ICF.

Abbreviations: HCO_3^-, bicarbonate; PCO_2, partial pressure of carbon dioxide; GI, gastrointestinal; NaHCO$_3$, sodium bicarbonate; PN, parenteral nutrition; H^+, hydrogen; ECF, extracellular fluid; ICF, intracellular fluid.
[a]Evaluation of urine chloride is sometimes used to aid in diagnosis. A low-urine chloride (<10 mmol/L) is found in chloride-responsive alkalosis and a high-urine chloride (>20 mmol/L) is consistent with chloride-unresponsive alkalosis.

Table 6.23   Expected Compensation, Causes, and Treatment of Respiratory Acidosis

Uncompensated or acute <24 hours
- Low pH (<7.35)
- High PCO_2 (>45 mmHg = hypercapnia)
- Normal or slightly increased HCO_3^- ($\geq$21–28 mEq/L)

Compensated or chronic
- Near normal pH
- High PCO_2
- High HCO_3^-
- Renal compensation occurs by the excretion of chloride and retaining HCO_3^-. HCO_3^- rises approximately 3–4 mEq/L for each 10-mmHg increase in PCO_2.

Principal causes
- Hypoventilation with inadequate excretion of CO_2
- Respiratory center depression:
  - Anesthesia
  - Brain injury or tumor
  - Drug overdose (sedative, barbiturate)
  - Pickwickian syndrome
  - Primary hypoventilation
- Restrictive defects:
  - Flail chest
  - Hemothorax or pneumothorax
  - Pneumonia
  - Kyphoscoliosis
  - Obesity
- Neuromuscular abnormalities:
  - Brain stem injury
  - Myasthenia gravis, Guillain-Barré syndrome, multiple sclerosis, muscular dystrophy, or amyotrophic lateral sclerosis
  - Diaphragmatic paralysis
- Airway obstruction:
  - Aspiration
  - Bronchospasm
  - Sleep apnea
  - Obstructive lung disease (bronchitis, emphysema)

(continued)

Table 6.23   Expected Compensation, Causes, and Treatment of Respiratory Acidosis (continued)

- Respiratory/circulatory collapse:
  - Cardiac arrest
  - Severe pulmonary edema
  - Pulmonary embolism

Treatment

- Correct underlying disturbance.
- Supplement oxygen or mechanical ventilation as needed.
- Overfeeding, especially of carbohydrate, resulting in excess CO_2 production can exacerbate an acute respiratory acidosis. Calories should be limited to maintenance requirements.

Abbreviations: PCO_2, partial pressure of carbon dioxide; HCO_3^-, bicarbonate; CO_2, carbon dioxide.

Table 6.24   Expected Compensation, Causes, and Treatment of Respiratory Alkalosis

Uncompensated or acute <24 hours

- High pH (>7.45)
- Low PCO_2 (<35 mmHg = hypocapnia)
- Normal HCO_3^- (21–28 mEq/L)

Compensated or chronic

- Near normal pH
- Low PCO_2
- Low HCO_3^-
- Renal compensation occurs through reabsorption of chloride and HCO_3^- excretion. HCO_3^- decreases approximately 4–6 mEq/L for each 10-mmHg decrease in PCO_2.

Principal causes

- Hyperventilation with excess elimination of CO_2
- Mechanical overventilation
- Central nervous system–mediated:
  - Voluntary hyperventilation (anxiety, hysteria)
  - Pain
  - Brain trauma or tumor
  - Cerebrovascular accident

(continued)

Table 6.24   Expected Compensation, Causes, and Treatment of Respiratory Alkalosis (continued)

- Hypoxemia or tissue hypoxia:
  - High altitude
  - Severe anemia
- Pulmonary diseases:
  - Pneumonia
  - Pulmonary embolism
  - Pulmonary edema
  - Interstitial lung disease
  - Early acute respiratory distress syndrome
- Pregnancy
- Hepatic failure
- Gram-negative sepsis
- Salicylate overdose

Treatment
- Correct underlying disturbance.
- Maintain adequate oxygenation.

Abbreviations: PCO_2, partial pressure of carbon dioxide; HCO_3^-, bicarbonate; CO_2, carbon dioxide.

HYDRATION AND LABORATORY VALUES

Analysis of several blood and urine indexes can offer insight into a patient's hydration status, although none will accurately predict the degree of volume deficit or excess. Interpretation requires knowledge of disease states, acid-base imbalances, and concurrent therapies that also influence laboratory results. Laboratory assessment is then used to support findings from the history and physical examination that correlate with volume depletion or excess (see Chapter 5). For more information on laboratory assessment and hydration status, see references 15, 16, 18, 19, 20, and 21.

The fluid content of the body is mainly found in the ICF and ECF compartments, with a small amount of transcellular fluid within specialized cavities. The ECF is further divided into fluid within the intravascular (blood vessels) and extravascular (interstitial) spaces.

Hypovolemia

Hypovolemia, or true volume depletion, refers to a loss of water and sodium leading to ECF volume contraction. In contrast, *dehydration* refers to the clinical consequences resulting from excessive loss of free water.

- Elevated blood urea nitrogen (BUN) may suggest hypovolemia, especially if a disproportionate rise relative to creatinine is seen by a BUN-to-creatinine ratio that exceeds 20:1 (and other causes such as excessive protein intake or GI bleeding are ruled out).
- Hypovolemia resulting in decreased intravascular fluid causes hemoconcentration. The relative fluctuations in hematocrit and albumin due to intravascular plasma volume changes must be compared with the patient's baseline values.
- Serum sodium and osmolality are nonspecific and have the least clinical utility when viewed in isolation.
- Urine-specific gravity and osmolality reflect the ability of the kidneys to concentrate or dilute urine appropriately and can provide additional information when assessing hydration status.

Hypervolemia

Hypervolemia is a state of ECF volume expansion. Compared with hypovolemia, laboratory indexes are even less specific for volume changes in this condition.

*Specific Laboratory Values Associated
with Hydration Status*

See Table 6.25 for additional information on using laboratory values to assess hydration status.

Table 6.25   Selected Laboratory Values and Hydration Status

BUN and BUN-to-creatinine ratio
- Normal:
  - BUN 10–20 mg/dL
  - BUN:creatinine ratio 10–15:1
- Hypovolemia: Increases
- Hypervolemia: Decreases
- Other factors associated with *low* lab values:
  - Inadequate dietary protein
  - Severe liver failure
- Other factors associated with *high* lab values:
  - Prerenal failure
  - Excessive protein intake
  - GI bleeding
  - Catabolic state
  - Glucocorticoid therapy
  - Creatinine also rises in severe hypovolemia.

Hematocrit
- Normal:
  - Males: 42%–52%
  - Females: 37%–47%
- Hypovolemia: Increases
- Hypervolemia: Decreases
- Other factors associated with *low* lab values:
  - Anemia
  - Hemorrhage with subsequent hemodilution (occurring after approximately 12–24 h)
- Other factors associated with *high* lab values:
  - Chronic hypoxia (chronic pulmonary disease, living at high altitude, heavy smoking)
  - Polycythemia vera
  - Recent transfusion

(continued)

Table 6.25   Selected Laboratory Values and Hydration Status
(continued)

Serum albumin
- Normal: 3.5–5 g/dL
- Hypovolemia: Increases
- Hypervolemia: Decreases
- Other factors influencing lab results:
  ○ Refer to the Serum Protein section of this chapter.
  ○ High levels are uncommon except in hemoconcentration.

Serum sodium
- Normal: 136–145 mEq/L
- Hypovolemia: Typically increases (but can be normal or decreased)
- Hypervolemia: Decreases, normal, or increases
- Other factors influencing lab results:
  ○ Refer to Hyponatremia and Hypernatremia in the Electrolyte Assessment section of this chapter.

Serum osmolality
- Normal: 285–295 mOsm/kg H_2O
- Hypovolemia: Typically increases, but can be decreased or normal
- Hypervolemia: Typically decreases, but can be increased or normal
- Other factors influencing lab results:
  ○ Refer to Hyponatremia and Hypernatremia in the Electrolyte Assessment section of this chapter.

Urine-specific gravity
- Normal (random): 1.003–1.03
- Hypovolemia: Increases
- Hypervolemia: Decreases
- Other factors associated with *low* lab values:
  ○ Renal disease
  ○ Diuresis
  ○ Diabetes insipidus in the elderly due to impaired ability to concentrate urine
- Other factors associated with *high* lab values:
  ○ Glucosuria
  ○ Proteinuria
  ○ Excretion of radiopaque dyes

(continued)

Table 6.25   Selected Laboratory Values and Hydration Status
(continued)

Urine osmolality
- Normal: 200–1200 mOsm/kg H_2O
- Hypovolemia: Increases
- Hypervolemia: Decreases
- Other factors associated with *low* lab values:
  - Diuresis (osmolality decreases as urine output increases, and vice versa)
  - Diabetes insipidus
  - Glomerulonephritis
  - Hyponatremia
  - Sickle cell anemia
  - Aldosteronism
- Other factors associated with *high* lab values:
  - Addison disease
  - Azotemia
  - Cirrhosis
  - Glucosuria
  - SIADH

Abbreviations: BUN, blood urea nitrogen; GI, gastrointestinal; H_2O, water; SIADH, syndrome of inappropriate antidiuretic hormone.

NUTRITIONAL ANEMIA ASSESSMENT

Nutritional anemias are most commonly caused by inadequate red blood cell (RBC) production due to a deficiency of iron, vitamin B-12, or folate. Laboratory values progressively change as the severity of anemia increases, with reduced hemoglobin (< 14 g/dL in men; < 12 g/dL in women) appearing in the later stages of nutrient depletion. For more information on topics addressed in this section, see references 3, 15, 16, and 25–29.

A number of laboratory tests, along with medical and nutrition histories, are useful for detection of early deficiency and to increase the diagnostic specificity. Within one or two weeks after starting effective replacement therapy to correct a vitamin B-12-deficiency anemia, folate-deficiency anemia, or iron-deficiency anemia, an increased reticulocyte count would be expected because increased RBCs are produced in response to therapy.

Iron-Deficiency Anemia (IDA) and Anemia of Chronic Disease (ACD)

Although iron deficiency is the most common cause of anemia worldwide, anemia of chronic disease (ACD) may be more prevalent in the hospital setting. Several hematologic features are similar (eg, a reduced serum iron and hemoglobin (Hgb), although Hgb rarely drops below 8 mg/dL in ACD). Their treatments vary, however, so it is important to distinguish between these two anemias.

The presence of anemia cannot be accurately diagnosed by clinical presentation alone, therefore laboratory assessment is required. Multiple blood tests (see Table 6.26) are commonly interpreted in conjunction with a nutrition and medical history (29). During an acute-phase response, iron studies are altered, which must be considered when interpreting the results. If blood tests are inconclusive, a bone marrow biopsy remains the gold standard for evaluating iron stores.

Table 6.26   Most Useful Laboratory Indexes for Diagnosis of Iron-Deficiency Anemia and Anemia of Chronic Disease[a]

Serum ferritin
- Normal:
  - Men: 12–300 ng/mL
  - Women: 10–150 ng/mL
- IDA: Decreases
- ACD: Normal or increases

Interpretation of laboratory tests:
- Serum ferritin reflects total-body iron stores.

(continued)

Table 6.26   Most Useful Laboratory Indexes for Diagnosis of Iron-Deficiency Anemia and Anemia of Chronic Disease[a] (continued)

- Serum ferritin < 10 ng/100 is considered diagnostic of iron deficiency and differentiates it from ACD.
- However, a normal ferritin level does not exclude iron deficiency because ferritin levels are increased with an acute-phase response, liver disease, renal disease, and some cancers.
- Excess levels are a sign of iron excess as in hemochromatosis, iron poisoning or recent blood transfusion.

Serum iron
- Normal:
  ○ Men: 80–180 mcg/dL
  ○ Women: 60–160 mcg/dL
- IDA: Decreases
- ACD: Decreases

Interpretation of laboratory tests:
- Serum iron represents the amount of iron in the blood where it is bound to transferrin and therefore available for RBC production.
- Levels are reduced in both IDA and ACD, although more markedly in severe IDA.
- Increases are observed in hemolytic states, hemachromatosis, iron overload, acute liver damage, and, transiently, after iron supplementation.
- Significant diurnal variation affects interpretation.

Total iron-binding capacity
- Normal: 250–460 mcg/dL
- IDA: Increases
- ACD: Decreases or low-normal

Interpretation of laboratory tests:
- TIBC is an indirect measurement of serum transferrin and reflects the amount of transferrin receptors available for iron binding.
- A rise in TIBC above normal is typically seen in iron deficiency, as well as, blood loss, acute liver damage, and late in pregnancy.
- However because transferrin is a negative acute-phase protein, it falls in any inflammatory state, even in the presence of iron deficiency (refer to Table 6.2).

(continued)

Table 6.26   Most Useful Laboratory Indexes for Diagnosis of Iron-Deficiency Anemia and Anemia of Chronic Disease[a] (continued)

Transferrin saturation
- Normal:
  - Men: 20%–50%
  - Women: 15%–50%
- IDA: Decreases (<16%–18%)
- ACD: Normal or low-normal (<20%)

Interpretation of laboratory tests:
- Transferrin saturation indicates the extent to which transferrin is saturated with iron and, therefore, the amount of iron available to the tissues.
- Decreases can be seen in both IDA and ACD, but more consistently and significantly in IDA.
- Transferrin saturation can be calculated by (serum iron × 100%) divided by TIBC.

Red cell distribution width
- Normal: 11%–14.5%
- IDA: Normal
- ACD: Increases

Interpretation of laboratory tests:
- Although nonspecific, an increased RDW can be a clue for evaluation of iron deficiency.
- RDW begins to rise relatively early in iron deficiency, typically before a decrease in mean corpuscular volume (MCV) is observed.
- However, it remains normal, or near normal, in ACD.

Mean corpuscular volume
- Normal: 80–95 fL
- IDA: Decreases
- ACD: Usually normal

Interpretation of laboratory tests:
- MCV measures the average size of RBCs.
- It is normal in early iron deficiency, then falls as anemia progresses.
- However, its diagnostic value is limited because reduced levels are also seen in approximately 15%–25% of patients with ACD.

(continued)

Table 6.26   Most Useful Laboratory Indexes for Diagnosis of Iron-Deficiency Anemia and Anemia of Chronic Disease[a] (continued)

Soluble transferrin receptor
- Normal: Range depends on assay used
- IDA: Increases
- ACD: Normal

Interpretation of laboratory tests:
- Useful to distinguish between IDA and ACD.
- Increased values seen in iron deficiency, hemolytic and megaloblastic anemias; myelodysplastic syndromes, and individuals living at high altitude or receiving erythropoietin therapy.

Abbreviations: IDA, iron-deficiency anemia; ACD, anemia of chronic disease; RBC, red blood cell; TIBC, total iron-binding capacity; RDW, red cell distribution width; MCV, mean corpuscular volume; TfR, transferrin receptor.
[a]ACD is an inability to use iron stores. It is typically mild and has a gradual onset, after a malignant, infectious, inflammatory or autoimmune condition. Therapy for ACD involves correcting the underlying disorder and use of erythropoietic agents. Iron supplementation is not beneficial unless a concurrent iron deficiency is present or if erythropoietin is used when the subsequent increase in RBC production requires supplemental iron. During critical illness, iron supplementation is recommended only with caution due to an increased risk of some infections.
Source: Data are from reference 29.

Vitamin B-12-Deficiency Anemia and Folate-Deficiency (Megaloblastic) Anemias

The presence of hypersegmented neutrophils on the peripheral blood smear, followed by an increased MCV, is an indication of vitamin B-12 or folate deficiency. However, many patients with vitamin B-12 deficiency develop neurologic and/or psychiatric symptoms before megaloblastic anemia manifests.

Serum or RBC folate and serum B-12 are commonly assessed simultaneously in an initial workup for suspected megaloblastic anemia. It is important to determine the cause of megaloblastic anemia because providing folic acid supplementation to a patient with B-12 deficiency will result in a transient improvement in the hematologic indexes but will allow any associated neurologic deterioration to continue. See Table 6.27 for additional information on laboratory assessment of these forms of anemia.

Table 6.27   Most Useful Laboratory Indexes for Diagnosis of Vitamin B-12-Deficiency Anemia and Folate-Deficiency Anemias

Mean corpuscular volume
- Normal: 80–95 fL
- Vitamin B-12-deficiency anemia: Increases
- Folate-deficiency anemia: Increases

Interpretation of laboratory tests:
- Evaluation of the MCV alone lacks sensitivity/specificity for megaloblastic anemia because elevations are also seen with alcoholism, liver disease, hypothyroidism, several medications, and some myelodysplastic disorders.
- Megaloblastic anemia is more likely if MCV is markedly elevated (> 110 fL); however, it can be normal with concurrent iron deficiency.

Serum B-12 (cobalamin)
- Normal: 160–950 pg/mL
- Vitamin B-12-deficiency anemia: Decreases
- Folate-deficiency anemia: Usually normal

Interpretation of laboratory tests:
- Interpretation of serum B-12 can be difficult because blood levels are maintained at the expense of tissue stores and a specific cutoff for deficiency is controversial.
- For unclear reasons, up to one-third of patients with folate deficiencies also have a decreased serum B-12, which rises with folate supplementation.

Serum methylmalonic acid
- Normal: 73–271 nmol/L
- Vitamin B-12-deficiency anemia: Increases
- Folate-deficiency anemia: Normal

Interpretation of laboratory tests:
- An elevated serum MMA is very specific for vitamin B-12 deficiency.
- However, increases can also be seen in dehydration or renal failure.
- Test availability is limited.

(continued)

Table 6.27   Most Useful Laboratory Indexes for Diagnosis of Vitamin B-12-Deficiency Anemia and Folate-Deficiency Anemias (continued)

Red blood cell folate
- Normal: 150–450 ng/mL
- Vitamin B-12-deficiency anemia: Normal or decreases
- Folate-deficiency anemia: Decreases

Interpretation of laboratory tests:
- RBC folate reflects folate adequacy during the previous 1–3 mo.
- However, the test has analytic limitations and levels are reduced in patients with folate deficiency and in about 50% of patients with B-12 deficiency (because cellular uptake of folate depends on B-12).

Serum folate
- Normal: 5–25 ng/mL
- Vitamin B-12-deficiency anemia: Normal or increases
- Folate-deficiency anemia: Decreases

Interpretation of laboratory tests:
- Measurement of serum folate is common, although it may be misleading because levels fluctuate rapidly with changes in recent dietary intake.
- A low folate level in both plasma and RBCs is a strong indicator of deficiency.

Serum homocysteine
- Normal: 4–14 mcmol/L
- Vitamin B-12-deficiency anemia: Increases greatly
- Folate-deficiency anemia: Increases moderately

Interpretation of laboratory tests:
- Increased serum homocysteine levels can be helpful but are nonspecific because elevations are seen in folate, B-12, and B-6 deficiency or, less frequently, in renal insufficiency, hypothyroidism, and several inherited disorders or some medications.

Abbreviations: MCV, mean corpuscular volume; MMA, methylmalonic acid; RBC, red blood cell.

VITAMIN, MINERAL, AND TRACE ELEMENT ASSESSMENT

Laboratory assessment can be useful to detect a subclinical nutrient deficiency or excess before physical signs manifest with some, but not all, micronutrients. An inadequate diet usually results in suboptimal status of several nutrients. However, isolated vitamin, mineral, or trace-element deficiencies can be the result of a disease state, medication interaction, or omission from PN. For more information on laboratory assessment of micronutrients, see references 15, 16, and 30–33.

Inadequate iron, vitamin B-12, folic acid, and thiamin may be relatively common in developed countries; in developing countries, however, vitamin A, zinc, iron, and iodine are among the most commonly seen deficiencies. Recent National Health and Nutrition Examination survey data report a decline in mean 25(OH)-vitamin D concentrations and using current cutoff points the prevalence of low vitamin D status seems to be growing worldwide (34).

The registered dietitian nutritionist (RDN) must be able to determine when laboratory assessment is warranted. Frequently, laboratory values can be misleading. Therefore, a thorough medical history, physical assessment, nutrition assessment, diet history, and knowledge of typical body nutrient stores are required to determine the likelihood of nutrient deficiency or excess. All sources of nutrients should be considered, including those found in lipid emulsions (intravenous lipid emulsions contain vitamin K as well as small amounts of phosphorus and vitamin E) and those synthesized by the body (vitamin K, biotin, and pantothenic acid from intestinal flora; vitamin D from sunlight; or niacin from tryptophan conversion).

The specific test and reference standards will vary with each laboratory's assay techniques. Interpretation can often be challenging because results can be altered by many nonnutritional factors, notably the acute phase response (see Tables 6.28–6.48).

Table 6.28   Laboratory Assessment of Vitamin A

Factors that cause or contribute to deficiency
- Fat malabsorption[a]
- Increased needs (burn, trauma, major surgery, infection)
- Medications (oral neomycin)

Recommended laboratory tests and interpretation
- Serum retinol:
  - May reflect long-term vitamin A status; plasma levels are maintained until liver reserves are nearly exhausted.
  - Decreases may also be seen in the acute-phase response, severe malnutrition, or zinc deficiency.
  - Renal failure and oral contraceptive use may increase levels.
  - Levels > 100 mcg/dL (>3.5 mcmol/L) are commonly seen in toxicity.
- Serum retinol-binding protein (a surrogate marker for retinol):
  - Concentrations are low in vitamin A deficiency, hyperthyroidism, chronic liver disorders, an acute-phase response, and cystic fibrosis.
  - Elevated levels occur in renal failure and acute or early liver damage.

[a]Malabsorption of fat-soluble vitamins can occur with inadequate pancreatic enzymes (chronic pancreatitis, cystic fibrosis), insufficient bile salts (biliary obstruction, cholestatic liver disease), short bowel syndrome, celiac disease, Crohn's disease, tropical sprue, and medications (cholestyramine, colestipol, mineral oil, and orlistat).

Table 6.29   Laboratory Assessment of Vitamin D

Factors that cause or contribute to deficiency
- Inadequate diet and/or inadequate skin exposure to ultraviolet light (eg, elderly or homebound individuals, especially in the winter)
- Renal or liver failure
- Nephrotic syndrome
- Hypoparathyroidism

(continued)

Table 6.29   Laboratory Assessment of Vitamin D (continued)

- Obesity
- Fat malabsorption[a]
- Gastrectomy
- Bariatric surgical procedures
- Medications:
  - Anticonvulsants[b] [especially if ≥2 agents]
  - Cimetidine
  - Isoniazid
  - Corticosteroids
  - Human immunodeficiency virus treatment medications

Recommended laboratory tests and interpretation
- Serum 25-hydroxyvitamin D:
  - Requires adequate liver function for synthesis
  - Concentrations vary with the season, sun exposure, and vitamin D intake.
  - Values <30 ng/mL are considered insufficient, whereas values <20ng/mL are classified as deficient.
  - Safe upper limit is 100 ng/mL.
- Serum 1,25-dihydroxyvitamin D:
  - Synthesis requires adequate renal function and supply of 25-hydroxyvitamin D.
  - Levels are typically low in deficiency; although occasionally normal as PTH, serum calcium, and phosphate levels closely regulate production of $1,25(OH)_2$.
  - Levels are normal or elevated in toxicity.
- Decreased serum phosphate and increased alkaline phosphatase and PTH are commonly seen in vitamin D deficiency; however, they are nonspecific for the diagnosis of vitamin D deficiency.

Abbreviation: PTH, parathyroid hormone.

[a]Malabsorption of fat-soluble vitamins can occur with inadequate pancreatic enzymes (chronic pancreatitis, cystic fibrosis), insufficient bile salts (biliary obstruction, cholestatic liver disease), short bowel syndrome, celiac disease, Crohn's disease, tropical sprue, and medications (cholestyramine, colestipol, mineral oil, and orlistat).

[b]Common anticonvulsants include phenobarbital, phenytoin, carbamazepine, and primidone.

Table 6.30   Laboratory Assessment of Vitamin E

Factors that cause or contribute to deficiency:
- Fat malabsorption[a]
- Abetalipoproteinemia
- Increased requirements with diets very high in polyunsaturated fats

Recommended laboratory tests and interpretation
- Plasma alpha tocopherol:
  - As vitamin E is transported in lipoproteins, interpretation requires an evaluation of lipid levels.
  - If hyperlipidemia is present, use an alpha tocopherol-to-lipid ratio. Plasma alpha-tocopherol-to-cholesterol (mmol/L) ratio <2.2 indicates a risk of vitamin E deficiency.

[a]Malabsorption of fat-soluble vitamins can occur with inadequate pancreatic enzymes (chronic pancreatitis, cystic fibrosis), insufficient bile salts (biliary obstruction, cholestatic liver disease), short bowel syndrome, celiac disease, Crohn's disease, tropical sprue, and medications (cholestyramine, colestipol, mineral oil, and orlistat).

Table 6.31   Laboratory Assessment of Vitamin K

Factors that cause or contribute to deficiency
- Fat malabsorption[a]
- Liver disease (primary biliary cirrhosis)
- Long-term PN without adequate vitamin K
- Medications:
  - Warfarin anticoagulants (an intentional effect)
  - Antibiotics (especially broad-spectrum and N-methylthiotetrazole–containing cephalosporins)
  - Megadoses of vitamin E
  - Anticonvulsants
  - High-dose aspirin
  - Quinine
  - Quinidine
  - Cyclosporine

(continued)

Table 6.31   Laboratory Assessment of Vitamin K (continued)

Recommended laboratory tests and interpretation
- PT:
  - A measure of blood clotting, PT is prolonged in vitamin K deficiency.
  - However, PT is insensitive to detect subclinical deficiency unless it rapidly normalizes (beginning within hours) after IV supplementation.
- Plasma phylloquinone (K_1):
  - Reflects recent dietary intake
  - Increased concentrations may be seen in older age and patients with hypertriglyceridemia.

Abbreviations: PN, parenteral nutrition; PT, prothrombin time; IV, intravenous.
[a]Malabsorption of fat-soluble vitamins can occur with inadequate pancreatic enzymes (chronic pancreatitis, cystic fibrosis), insufficient bile salts (biliary obstruction, cholestatic liver disease), short bowel syndrome, celiac disease, Crohn's disease, tropical sprue, and medications (cholestyramine, colestipol, mineral oil, and orlistat).

Table 6.32   Laboratory Assessment of Vitamin C

Factors that cause or contribute to deficiency
- Inadequate diet
- Increased requirements:
  - Trauma, burns
  - Chronic infection or inflammatory diseases
  - Smoking
  - Pregnancy or lactation
  - Hyperthyroidism
- Dialysis
- Medications:
  - Barbiturates
  - Tetracycline
  - High-dose aspirin

Recommended laboratory tests and interpretation
- Plasma ascorbic acid:
  - Reflects recent intake
  - The upper limit of 1.7 mg/dL is considered the renal threshold.
- Leukocyte ascorbic acid: Reflects tissue stores but is more technically difficult to perform and interpret

Table 6.33   Laboratory Assessment of Thiamin (Vitamin B-1)

Factors that cause or contribute to deficiency
- Alcoholism (most common cause)
- Refeeding syndrome
- Inadequate diet or omission from PN (eg, during multivitamin shortage)
- Increased requirements:
  ○ Fever
  ○ Pregnancy or lactation
  ○ Hypermetabolism
  ○ Hyperthyroidism
- Dialysis
- Medications:
  ○ High-dose diuretics
  ○ Prolonged antacid use

Recommended laboratory tests and interpretation
- ETKA:
  ○ Can be used alone but is most sensitive/specific when thiamin pyrophosphate is added and interpreted along with a percentage of stimulation effect (TPPE)
  ○ The higher the percentage stimulation (or activity coefficient), the greater the deficiency
  ○ A delay to process test results can limit its usefulness when deciding whether prompt supplementation is warranted.
- Urinary thiamin:
  ○ Reflects recent intake
  ○ Requires an adequate renal conservation mechanism that decreases urinary excretion when body stores are depleted
- Increased serum lactate (lactic acidosis):
  ○ A nonspecific sign of thiamin deficiency

Abbreviations: PN, parenteral nutrition; ETKA, erythrocyte transketolase activity; TPPE, thiamin pyrophosphate effect.

Table 6.34   Laboratory Assessment of Riboflavin (Vitamin B-2)

Factors that cause or contribute to deficiency
- Inadequate diet
- Alcoholism
- Being elderly

(continued)

6.34   Laboratory Assessment of Riboflavin (Vitamin B-2)
(continued)

- Malabsorption: Celiac disease, tropical sprue
- Liver disease
- Biliary obstruction
- Hypothyroidism
- Diabetes mellitus
- Increased requirements:
  - Surgery
  - Trauma or burns
  - Pregnancy or lactation
- Medications:
  - Phenothiazines or tricyclic antidepressants (imipramine, amitriptyline)
  - Probenecid
  - Chlorpromazine
  - Adriamycin
  - Quinacrine

Recommended laboratory tests and interpretation:
- EGR-AC: A functional test reflecting riboflavin status

Abbreviation: EGR-AC, erythrocyte glutathione reductase activity coefficient.

Table 6.35   Laboratory Assessment of Niacin (Vitamin B-3)

Factors that cause or contribute to deficiency
- Alcoholism
- Carcinoid syndrome
- Hartnup's disease
- Malabsorption: Crohn's disease
- Medications:
  - Isoniazid
  - Mercaptopurine
- Increased requirements can occur in cirrhosis, hypermetabolism, burns, hyperthyroidism, diabetes mellitus, pregnancy and lactation, but they rarely result in a deficient state.

(continued)

Table 6.35   Laboratory Assessment of Niacin (Vitamin B-3)
(continued)

Recommended laboratory tests and interpretation
- Excretion of niacin metabolites in the urine is most commonly measured. Urinary 2-pyridone falls more precipitously than urinary N'-methylnicotinamide.
- A ratio is used if only a random urine specimen is available.

**Table 6.36   Laboratory Assessment of Panothenic Acid
(Vitamin B-5)**

Factors that cause or contribute to deficiency
- Severe prolonged malnutrition
- Alcoholism
- Deficiency is rare and would not occur as an isolated deficiency.

Recommended laboratory tests and interpretation
- Urinary pantothenic acid (24 h): Closely related to dietary intake but varies greatly among individuals.

Table 6.37   Laboratory Assessment of Pyridoxine (Vitamin B-6)

Factors that cause or contribute to deficiency
- Alcoholism
- Liver disease
- Inadequate diet
- Severe riboflavin deficiency
- Medications:
  ◦ Isoniazid
  ◦ Hydralazine
  ◦ Cycloserine
  ◦ Penicillamine
  ◦ Possibly oral contraceptives
- Increased requirements:
  ◦ Chronic renal failure, dialysis
  ◦ Pregnancy, eclampsia, preeclampsia

(continued)

Table 6.37   Laboratory Assessment of Pyridoxine (Vitamin B-6) (continued)

Recommended laboratory tests and interpretation
- Plasma pyridoxal 5'-phosphate (PLP): Interpretation is challenging because it is influenced by many factors, including exercise, pregnancy, age, alkaline phosphatase levels, smoking, and some medications.

Table 6.38   Laboratory Assessment of Folic Acid

Factors that cause or contribute to deficiency
- Inadequate diet
- Alcoholism
- Increased requirements:
  - Pregnancy or lactation
  - Hemolytic anemia
  - Chronic exfoliative dermatitis
  - Dialysis
- Being elderly
- Malabsorption:
  - Short bowel syndrome
  - Celiac disease
  - Tropical sprue
- Medications:
  - Sulfasalazine
  - Folic acid antagonists[a]
  - Pentamidine
  - Triamterene
  - Piritrexim
  - Epoetin
  - Anticonvulsants[b] (although large folic acid supplementation may reverse their effectiveness)
  - Cycloserine
  - Possibly oral contraceptives

Recommended laboratory tests and interpretation
- Serum folate:
  - Indicates recent dietary intake and may not correlate with tissue stores
  - May be elevated in vitamin B-12 deficiency or intestinal bacterial overgrowth

(continued)

Table 6.38   Laboratory Assessment of Folic Acid (continued)

- Erythrocyte (RBC) folate:
  - Reflects intake for the life of the RBC (120 d)
- Simultaneous evaluation of Vitamin B-12 and homocysteine is recommended.
- Refer to the Anemia section of this chapter for more information.

Abbreviation: RBC, red blood cell.

[a]Folate antagonists (methotrexate, pyrimethamine, trimetrexate, trimethoprim) inhibit dihydrofolate reductase inhibitors and may result in folic acid deficiency.

[b]Common anticonvulsants include phenobarbital, phenytoin, carbamazepine, and primidone.

Table 6.39   Laboratory Assessment of Vitamin B-12

Factors that cause or contribute to deficiency
- Inadequate stomach acid:
  - Achlorhydria
  - Autoimmune atrophic gastritis, common in adults age ≥ 50 y
- Inadequate intrinsic factor:
  - Pernicious anemia
  - Gastrectomy or gastric bypass
- Resection or disease of the terminal ileum:
  - Short bowel syndrome
  - Blind loop syndrome
  - Tropical sprue
- Vegan diet
- AIDS
- Medications:
  - Proton pump inhibitors[a]
  - H_2 blockers[b]
  - Neomycin
  - Colchicine
  - p-aminosalicylic acid
  - Nitrous oxide
  - Metformin
  - Cholestyramine
  - Epoetin
  - Anticonvulsants

(continued)

Table 6.39   Laboratory Assessment of Vitamin B-12 (continued)

Recommended laboratory tests and interpretation
- Serum cobalamin (B-12):
  ○ Most commonly used method; however, levels may be maintained at the expense of tissue stores.
  ○ Elevations (including falsely high levels) can occur in myeloproliferative disorders (leukemia, lymphomas, polycythemia vera) and active liver disease.
- Serum MMA:
  ○ Increases early in B-12 deficiency but not in folate deficiency
- Simultaneous evaluation of folic acid and homocysteine is recommended.
- Refer to the Anemia section of this chapter for more information.

Abbreviations: H_2 blockers, histamine H_2-receptor antagonists; MMA, methylmalonic acid.
[a]Proton pump inhibitors include omeprazole and lansoprazole.
[b]H_2 blockers include cimetidine, ranitidine, and famotidine.

Table 6.40   Laboratory Assessment of Biotin

Factors that cause or contribute to deficiency
- PN without biotin, especially in short bowel syndrome
- Excessive/prolonged consumption of raw egg whites
- Chronic hemodialysis
- Medications: anticonvulsants
- Deficiency is rare as biotin is ubiquitous in the diet and produced by intestinal bacteria.

Recommended laboratory tests and interpretation
- Urinary biotin excretion:
  ○ Reduced in biotin deficiency
  ○ Testing is technically demanding, and interpretation is difficult.
- Urinary 3-hydroxisovalerate acid: increased in biotin deficiency

Abbreviation: PN, parenteral nutrition.

Table 6.41   Laboratory Assessment of Iron[a]

Factors that cause or contribute to deficiency
- Blood loss from GI tract:
  ○ Cancer
  ○ Inflammatory bowel disease
  ○ Ulcers
  ○ Hookworm
- Heavy menstruation
- Hemodialysis
- Increased requirements:
  ○ Pregnancy
  ○ Epoetin therapy
- Chronic renal failure
- Inadequate diet/vegetarian diet
- Long-term PN without iron
- Malabsorption:
  ○ Celiac disease
  ○ Crohn's disease
  ○ Short bowel syndrome
- Achlorhydria:
  ○ Atrophic gastritis
  ○ Gastrectomy or gastric bypass
- Medications:
  ○ Epoetin
  ○ Chronic aspirin use
  ○ Proton pump inhibitors[b]
  ○ H_2 blockers[c]

Recommended laboratory tests and interpretation
- Refer to Table 6.26 for additional information on testing for iron-deficiency anemia.
- Serum ferritin:
  ○ Falls with depletion of iron stores
  ○ Greatly elevated levels are seen in iron overload.
- Soluble TfR:
  ○ Rises early in iron deficiency and in proportion to the magnitude of the deficit
  ○ Can help to distinguish between iron deficiency and anemia of chronic disease

(continued)

6.41   Laboratory Assessment of Iron[a] (continued)

- ○ Results are not affected by the acute-phase response, pregnancy, age, or gender.
- ○ Test availability is limited.

Abbreviations: GI, gastrointestinal; PN, parenteral nutrition; H_2 blockers, histamine H_2-receptor antagonists; TfR, transferrin receptor.
[a]Iron is not routinely added to PN.
[b]Proton pump inhibitors include omeprazole and lansoprazole.
[c]H_2 blockers include cimetidine, ranitidine, and famotidine.

Table 6.42   Laboratory Assessment of Zinc

Factors that cause or contribute to deficiency
- Malabsorption:
  - ○ Celiac disease
  - ○ Crohn's disease
  - ○ Short bowel syndrome
  - ○ AIDS enteropathy
  - ○ Large-volume ileostomy, diarrhea, or enteric fistula output
- Increased renal losses:
  - ○ Chronic liver disease/cirrhosis
  - ○ Nephrotic syndrome
  - ○ Some cancers
  - ○ Diabetes
  - ○ Alcoholism
  - ○ Trauma
- PN without adequate zinc
- Inadequate diet: high-phytate/vegetarian
- Being elderly
- Burns
- Sickle cell anemia
- Acrodermatitis enteropathica
- Medications:
  - ○ Penicillamine
  - ○ Diuretics
  - ○ Diethylenetriamine penta-acetate
  - ○ Valproate

(continued)

6.42   Laboratory Assessment of Zinc (continued)

Recommended laboratory tests and interpretation
- Plasma zinc:
  - Interpret with caution.
  - Homeostatic mechanisms can maintain plasma concentrations for weeks despite inadequate intake.
  - Unreliable in acute illness as decreases also correlate with degree of hypoalbuminemia and redistribution in acute-phase response.
  - Assessment of zinc status based on hair analysis lacks clearly defined lower cutoff values.

Abbreviation: PN, parenteral nutrition.

Table 6.43   Laboratory Assessment of Copper

Factors that cause or contribute to deficiency
- PN without copper
- Increased losses:
  - Diarrhea
  - Enteric fistulas
  - Large burn wounds
  - Nephrotic syndrome
  - Abnormal bile loss
- Malabsorption:
  - Celiac disease
  - Short bowel syndrome
  - Tropical sprue
- PCM, especially recovery (although low serum levels may be due to low ceruloplasmin production)
- Medications:
  - Penicillamine
  - High-dose zinc or iron
- Deficiency is relatively rare.

(continued)

Table 6.43   Laboratory Assessment of Copper (continued)

Recommended laboratory tests and interpretation
- Plasma copper or ceruloplasmin:
  - \>90% of copper in plasma is bound to ceruloplasmin, and changes in blood levels are usually parallel.
  - Plasma copper is a reliable indicator of copper deficiency but does not reflect intake except when below a certain level.
  - May not be sensitive for marginal deficiency
  - Refer to age-specific and sex-specific ranges.
  - Values increase with pregnancy, malignancy, myocardial infarction, oral contraceptive use, or an acute-phase response (as ceruloplasmin is a positive acute-phase protein).
- Erythrocyte Cu/Zn superoxide dismutase:
  - Reflects long-term status
  - Not commonly used

Abbreviations: PN, parenteral nutrition; PCM, protein-calorie malnutrition; Cu, coppper; Zn, zinc.

Table 6.44   Laboratory Assessment of Selenium[a]

Factors that cause or contribute to deficiency
- Residence in areas with low-selenium soil (eg, China, New Zealand, Scandinavia)
- PN without selenium
- Malabsorption:
  - Prolonged diarrhea
  - Enteric fistulas
  - Crohn's disease, inflammatory bowel disease
  - Short bowel syndrome

Recommended laboratory tests and interpretation
- Plasma selenium:
  - The most commonly used index of selenium status
  - Under steady-state conditions, it reflects intake and selenium nutriture; however, correlation with total body stores has not been established.

Abbrevation: PN, parenteral nutrition.
[a]Selenium is available in some trace element packages.

Table 6.45   Laboratory Assessment of Chromium[a]

Factors that cause or contribute to deficiency
- Long-term PN without supplementation
- Requirement increased with large intestinal losses

Recommended laboratory tests and interpretation
- No reliable assay is widely available. Sample contamination is a problem.
- As glucose intolerance and elevated LDL cholesterol and triglycerides can be seen in chromium deficiency, improved levels after chromium supplementation have been used as an indirect indicator of chromium deficiency.

Abbreviations: PN, parenteral nutrition; LDL, low-density lipoprotein.
[a]Chromium is found as a contaminant of amino acid solutions in addition to the content in the trace element package.

Table 6.46   Laboratory Assessment of Manganese

Factors that cause or contribute to deficiency
- Deficiency is extremely rare (eg, clinical tests with purified diet).
- Toxicity has been reported in patients receiving PN, especially if biliary excretion is impaired by cholestatic disease.

Recommended laboratory tests and interpretation
- No sensitive and specific indicator
- Whole blood manganese:
  ◦ Correlates with MRI abnormalities and is often the most practical option
  ◦ However, results are highly variable.
- Plasma manganese:
  ◦ Assay has limited availability and is technically difficult.
  ◦ Sample contamination is a problem, and slight hemolysis of samples can markedly increase concentration.
- Erythrocyte manganese:
  ◦ May reflect tissue concentrations
  ◦ Assay is not widely available.
- Toxicity may be noted by elevated blood manganese or manganese deposition in the brain, observed on an MRI

Abbreviations: PN, parenteral nutrition; MRI, magnetic resonance imaging.

Table 6.47   Laboratory Assessment of Molybdenum[a]

Factors that cause or contribute to deficiency
- Rare genetic molybdenum cofactor deficiency
- One reported case on long-term PN with Crohn's disease
- Deficiency is extremely unlikely.

Recommended laboratory tests and interpretation
- Testing is difficult to perform and requires atomic absorption spectrophotometry or emission spectroscopy.
- Adequate assay and guidelines not available for nutrition assessment.

Abbreviation: PN, parenteral nutrition.
[a]Molybdenum is available in some trace element packages.

Table 6.48   Laboratory Assessment of Iodine[a]

Factors that cause or contribute to deficiency
- Inadequate diet in endemic areas or unsupplemented food supplies
- Increased requirement in cold environments, stress, and with antithyroid medications
- Excessive consumption of goiterogenic foods (eg, cabbage, rutabagas, broccoli, cauliflower, cassava) is usually not a clinically significant factor except with a coexisting iodine deficiency.

Recommended laboratory tests and interpretation
- Urinary iodine excretion:
  ○ Used in population studies
  ○ Reflects very recent intake. Ideally, obtain a 24–h urine sample.
  ○ If a random sample, compare to urinary creatinine.
  ○ An indirect measurement of iodine deficiency is a normal or low total T_4, normal or slightly elevated T_3, and a normal or only slightly elevated TSH.

Abbreviations: T_4, thyroxine; T_3, triiodothyronine; TSH, thyroid-stimulating hormone; PN, parenteral nutrition.
[a]Iodine is not routinely added to PN.

DISEASE-SPECIFIC LABORATORY TESTING
FOR ADULTS

Table 6.49 explains the use of stool studies (15,16,35,36) in adult patients. Tables 6.50 through 6.54 describe some key uses of laboratory testing used to monitor and evaluate factors related to each nutrition diagnosis and intervention implemented by the RDN. The tables are designed to illustrate laboratory testing often ordered for adult patients who either have or are at risk for:

- Chronic kidney disease (CKD)—see Table 6.50 (37–39)
- Refeeding syndrome—see Table 6.51 (3,40,41)
- Essential fatty acid deficiency (EFAD)—see Table 6.52 (42,43)
- Hyperlipidemia—see Table 6.53 (13,44,45)
- Metabolic syndrome—see Table 6.54 (46).
  - **Note**: Various criteria have been proposed for the diagnosis of metabolic syndrome by different organizations over the past decade. Despite an effort to harmonize the criteria for metabolic syndrome, differences persist in the criteria of waist circumference. A complete table on waist circumference criteria by organization, race, and gender is available in reference 46. Organizations agree on the parameters for laboratory values and that any three of five measures is diagnostic for metabolic syndrome.

Table 6.49   Stool Studies: Laboratory Tests, Frequency of Monitoring, and Rationale

Fecal leukocytes

- The presence of fecal leukocytes (white blood cells) is a screening test for infectious or inflammatory etiologies of acute diarrhea.
- Positive tests are seen with bacteria that penetrate intestinal mucosa, such as *Shigella*, *Salmonella*, *Escherichia coli*, and *Campylobacter*, as well as inflammatory processes such as ulcerative colitis and antibiotic-associated colitis.
- Fecal leukocytes will not be present in diarrhea due to noninvasive bacteria or due to viral or noninfectious causes.

Ova and parasites

- Diagnosis of parasitic infection is not common in hospitalized patients unless the patient has had recent foreign travel or children in day care.
- Positive results are also unlikely in nosocomial diarrhea (stool specimens submitted after 3 d of hospitalization).

***Clostridium difficile* toxin**

- *C. difficile*–associated diarrhea usually occurs within 1–2 mo of antibiotic use (especially clindamycin, cephalosporins, or penicillins) or occasionally chemotherapeutic agents. Diarrhea, abdominal cramps, tenderness, fever, and leukocytosis are common, although symptoms vary.
- Stool culture is the most sensitive test and involves a 2-step method that uses detection of GDH as initial screening and then uses the cell cytotoxicity assay or toxigenic culture as the confirmatory test for GDH-positive stool samples only. Repeat testing during the same episode of diarrhea is of limited value.
- Treatment typically includes metronidazole or oral vancomycin; antidiarrheal medications are avoided. Use of certain probiotics for prevention and treatment of antibiotic- and *C. difficile*–associated diarrhea may be beneficial.

Sudan stain test

- This qualitative screening test for fat malabsorption can use a random stool sample.
- Results are reported as normal (1+), slight increase (2+), and definite increase (3+) and are only reliable for moderate to severe steatorrhea.

(continued)

**Table 6.49   Stool Studies: Laboratory Tests, Frequency of
Monitoring, and Rationale** (continued)

Fecal fat
- A 72-h stool collection is obtained for a quantitative evaluation of steatorrhea. The patient should consume a diet containing 80–100 g fat/d for 1–2 days before and during the study period.
- <7 g fat per day (or 7%) is considered normal absorption.
- As a coefficient of fat absorption is calculated, the test requires an accurate record of dietary fat intake and a complete stool collection.

Fecal occult blood test
- Detection of occult blood in the stool suggests blood loss (eg, GI tumors, ulcerative colitis, regional enteritis, peptic ulcer, esophageal varices, or hemorrhoids).
- Red meat, vegetables (turnips, horseradish), and some medications (NSAIDs, iron) can cause false-positive results and vitamin C supplementation can cause false-negative results, depending on the test used.
- Serial testing is used because colorectal cancers may bleed intermittently.

Abbreviations: GDH, glutamate dehydrogenase; GI, gastrointestinal; NSAIDs, nonsteroidal anti-inflammatory drugs.
Source: Data are from references 15, 16, 35, and 36.

**Table 6.50   Chronic Kidney Disease: Laboratory Tests,
Frequency of Monitoring, and Rationale**

Albumin, prealbumin
- Regulatory agencies (eg, CMS) currently require monitoring of serum albumin as a marker of nutritional status in patients who have CKD. RDNs must use appropriate critical thinking skills in assessing nutritional status.
- Predialysis or stabilized[a] albumin should be measured monthly for maintenance dialysis (or every 1–3 months for nondialyzed patients with chronic renal failure), and prealbumin as needed.
- Goal:
  - Albumin ≥4 mg/dL (for the bromcresol green method)
  - Prealbumin ≥30 mg/dL
- The presence of acute or chronic inflammation limits the specificity of serum albumin or serum prealbumin as a nutritional marker.[b]

(continued)

**Table 6.50   Chronic Kidney Disease: Laboratory Tests,
Frequency of Monitoring, and Rationale** (continued)

Serum creatinine
- Patients with predialysis or stabilized serum creatinine
  < 10 mg/dL should be assessed for malnutrition and skeletal
  muscle wasting.
- A low serum creatinine concentration suggests low dietary
  protein intake and/or diminished skeletal muscle mass and is
  associated with increased mortality rates.

**Sodium, potassium, chloride, bicarbonate, calcium,
phosphorus**
- Used in the assessment of fluid and acid-base imbalances, or
  the need for dietary alteration
- Risk of soft-tissue deposition if serum calcium-phosphorus
  product exceeds 70 mg/dL; goal is < 55 mg^2/dL^2.
- Bicarbonate should be measured monthly, with predialysis or
  stabilized levels maintained ≥22 mmol/L.

Hemoglobin, CBC, transferrin saturation, serum ferritin
- Patients with CKD are at high risk of anemia due to inadequate
  erythropoietin and iron deficiency.
- Assess hemoglobin at least annually. If < 13.5 g/dL (males) or
  < 12 g/dL (females), obtain CBC, absolute reticulocyte count,
  ferritin, and transferrin saturation.
- Monitor hemoglobin (monthly) and iron status tests (every
  1–3 mo) during use of erythropoiesis-stimulating agents.

Fasting lipid profile
- Evaluate all patients with CKD for dyslipidemias (ie, risk of
  elevated TG, LDL, IDL, and VLDL, and decreased HDL).
- However, if total cholesterol is declining or low (< 150–180
  mg/dL), screening for malnutrition is recommended.

Intact PTH and 25-hydroxyvitamin D
- Patients with CKD should be screened for vitamin D
  insufficiency/deficiency.
- If intact PTH is above target range, obtain baseline
  25-hydroxyvitamin D measurement and, if normal, repeat
  annually.
- Algorithms for vitamin D supplementation are published
  elsewhere (38).

(continued)

Table 6.50   Chronic Kidney Disease: Laboratory Tests, Frequency of Monitoring, and Rationale (continued)

Aluminum
- To evaluate the risk of aluminum toxicity, obtain serum aluminum level at least annually, and every 3 months if receiving aluminum-containing medications.
- Goal: <20 mcg/L.

Abbreviations: CMS, Centers for Medicare & Medicaid Services; CKD, chronic kidney disease; RDN, registered dietitian nutritionist; CBC, complete blood count; TG, triglycerides; LDL, low-density lipoproteins; IDL, intermediate-density lipoproteins; VLDL, very low–density lipoproteins; HDL, high-density lipoproteins; PTH, parathyroid hormone.
[a]A predialysis measurement is obtained immediately before the initiation of a hemodialysis or intermittent peritoneal dialysis treatment. A stabilized serum measurement is obtained after the patient has stabilized on continuous ambulatory peritoneal dialysis.
[b]Refer to earlier discussion in the chapter regarding the utility of albumin measurement in inflammatory conditions.
Source: Data are from references 37–39.

Table 6.51   Risk of Refeeding Syndrome: Laboratory Tests, Frequency of Monitoring, and Rationale

Potassium, phosphorus, magnesium
- Initiating carbohydrate-rich nutrition after a period of starvation stimulates electrolytes to shift from the blood into the tissues for anabolism.
  - The hallmark of refeeding syndrome is hypophosphatemia, but the syndrome often includes sodium and fluid imbalances as well as hypokalemia and hypomagnesemia.
  - High-risk conditions include anorexia nervosa, alcoholism, cancer cachexia, prolonged hypocaloric feeding, and profound weight loss.
  - Baseline electrolyte concentrations are often normal, then rapidly decline upon initiation of feeding, or in some cases, electrolyte changes can be observed upon initiation of IVF containing dextrose.

(continued)

**Table 6.51   Risk of Refeeding Syndrome: Laboratory Tests,
Frequency of Monitoring, and Rationale** (continued)

- Take preventive actions:
  - Obtain and correct baseline electrolytes prior to initiation of nutrition support.
  - Nutrition support should be initiated at approximately 25% of the estimated goal.
  - Increase energy intake gradually.
  - Monitor electrolytes at least daily until stable at full caloric target (typically the first 3–5 d).

Abbreviation: IVF, intravenous fluid.
Source: Data are from references 3, 40, and 41.

**Table 6.52   Essential Fatty Acid Deficiency: Laboratory Tests,
Frequency of Monitoring, and Rationale**

Triene (eicosatrienoic acid)-to-tetraene (arachidonic acid) ratio
- Risk factors for EFAD include:
  - Severe fat malabsorption
  - Nutrition support containing <2%–4% of energy from linoleic acid and/or 0.25%–0.5% alpha linolenic acid.
- Biochemical signs of deficiency can occur within 2–4 weeks of fat-free EN or PN.
- Manifestation is delayed when a hypocaloric or cyclic regimen enables lipolysis of endogenous fat stores.
- Normal ratios in adults are 0.01–0.038. A triene-to-tetraene ratio of >0.4 suggests EFAD, with levels >0.2 confirming deficiency.
- This test is not often used in clinical practice because few labs process it, which delays results, and because the test is cost prohibitive.
- Clinicians should look for signs and symptoms during the physical assessment (see Chapter 5).
- A complete fatty acid profile can be obtained from several US laboratories using gas chromatography–mass spectrometry stable isotope dilution analysis.

Abbreviations: EFAD, essential fatty acid deficiency; EN, enteral nutrition; PN, parenteral nutrition.
Source: Data are from references 42 and 43.

Table 6.53   Hyperlipidemia: Laboratory Tests, Frequency of Monitoring, and Rationale

Fasting lipoprotein profile (total, LDL and HDL cholesterol, triglycerides)
- Screening for hyperlipidemia is recommended every 5 y for everyone aged ≥20 y.
- In most patients with diabetes, lipids should be measured at least annually; those younger than 40 years with a low-risk profile should have repeat assessments every 2 years.

Classification of lipid levels
- LDL-C:
  - <100 mg/dL is optimal.
  - 100–129 mg/dL is near or above optimal.
  - 130–159 is borderline high.
  - 160–189 mg/dL is high.
  - ≥190 mg/dL is very high.
- Total cholesterol:
  - <200 mg/dL is desirable.
  - 200–239 mg/dL is borderline high.
  - ≥240 mg/dL is high.
- HDL-C:
  - <40 mg/dL is low.
  - ≥60 mg/dL is high.
- TG:
  - <150 mg/dL is normal.
  - 150–199 mg/dL is borderline high.
  - 200–499 mg/dL is high.
  - ≥500 mg/dL is very high.

LDL-C goal
- High-risk patients:
  - <100 mg/dL
  - Optional goal is <70 mg/dL, especially if very high risk
- Moderately high-risk patients: <130 mg/dL
- Moderate-risk patients: <130 mg/dL
- Lower risk patients: <160 mg/dL

Abbreviations: LDL-C, low-density lipoprotein cholesterol; HDL-C, high-density lipoprotein cholesterol; TG, triglycerides.
Source: Data are from references 13, 43, and 44.

Table 6.54   Criteria for Clinical Diagnosis of Metabolic Syndrome

Measure	Categorical Cut Points
Elevated WC[a,b]	Population- and country-specific definitions
Elevated TG (Drug treatment for elevated TG is an alternate indicator.)[c]	≥150 mg/dL (1.7 mmol/L)
Reduced HDL-C (Drug treatment for reduced HDL-C is an alternate indicator.)[c]	<40 mg/dL (1 mmol/L) in males <50 mg/dL (1.3 mmol/L) in females
Elevated BP (Antihypertensive drug treatment in a patient with a history of hypertension is an alternate indicator.)	Systolic ≥130 mm Hg and/or diastolic ≥85 mm Hg
Elevated fasting glucose[d] (Drug treatment of elevated glucose is an alternate indicator.)	≥100 mg/dL

Abbreviations: WC, waist circumference; TG, triglycerides; HDL-C, high-density lipoprotein cholesterol; BP, blood pressure; IDF, International Diabetes Foundation; AHA, American Heart Association; NHLBI, National Heart, Lung, and Blood Institute.

[a]To measure WC, locate top of right iliac crest. Place a measuring tape in a horizontal plane around abdomen at level of iliac crest. Before reading tape measure, ensure that tape is snug but does not compress the skin and is parallel to floor. Measurement is made at the end of a normal expiration.

[b]It is recommended that the IDF cut points (≥94 cm in men, ≥80 cm in women) be used for non-Europeans and either the IDF or AHA/NHLBI cut points (≥102 cm in men, ≥88 cm in women) be used for people of European origin until more data are available.

[c]The most commonly used drugs for elevated TG and reduced HDL-C are fibrates and nicotinic acid. A patient taking one of these drugs can be presumed to have high TG and low HDL-C. High-dose omega-3 fatty acids presumes high triglycerides.

[d]Most patients with type 2 diabetes mellitus will have the metabolic syndrome by the proposed criteria.

Source: Adapted with permission from reference 46: Alberti KGMM, Eckel RH, Grundy SM, Zimmet PZ, Cleeman JI, Donato KA, Fruchart JC, James WP, Loria CM, Smith SC Jr. Harmonizing the metabolic syndrome: A joint interim statement of the International Diabetes Federation Task Force on Epidemiology and Prevention; National Heart, Lung, and Blood Institute; American Heart Association; World Heart Federation; International Atherosclerosis Society; and International Association for the Study of Obesity. *Circulation.* 2009;120:1640–1645. Copyright 2009 American Heart Association, Inc.

MONITORING DURING ENTERAL AND PARENTERAL NUTRITION

Frequency of monitoring and tests ordered should be individualized based on previous laboratory data, clinical condition, and underlying disease.

Monitoring in Acute Care Settings

Table 6.55 describes the frequency of monitoring required for selected laboratory tests used in critically ill and stable hospitalized patients (47,48).

Table 6.55   Acute Enteral Nutrition or Parenteral Nutrition: Laboratory Tests and Frequency of Monitoring

Laboratory Tests	Frequency of Monitoring[a]
Sodium, potassium, chloride, bicarbonate	• *Baseline and initiation:* Baseline; then daily for 3 d. More frequent monitoring may be needed with refeeding syndrome. • *Unstable or critically ill patients:* Daily • *Stable hospitalized patients:* 1–2 times/wk.
BUN, creatinine	• *Baseline and initiation:* Baseline; then daily for 3 d. • *Unstable or critically ill patients:* Daily. • *Stable hospitalized patients:* 1–2 times/wk.
Glucose	• *Baseline and initiation:* Baseline; then serum or finger stick every 8 h for the first 3 d; continue until consistently < 150 mg/dL. • *Unstable or critically ill patients:* Daily if < 150 mg/dL. Continue every 8 h if > 150 mg/dL. • *Stable hospitalized patients:* 1–2 times/wk if consistently < 150 mg/dL and not requiring insulin or oral agent. Continue every 8 h if > 150 mg/dL.

(continued)

Table 6.55 **Acute Enteral Nutrition or Parenteral Nutrition: Laboratory Tests and Frequency of Monitoring** (continued)

Calcium	• *Baseline and initiation:* Baseline, then daily for 3 d. If low, obtain ionized calcium before considering treatment. • *Unstable or critically ill patients:* Daily if unstable, otherwise 2–3 times/wk. • *Stable hospitalized patients:* 1–2 times/wk.
Phosphorus, magnesium	• *Baseline and initiation:* Baseline; then daily for 3 d. If low or risk of refeeding syndrome, monitor at least daily for 3 d or until consistently within normal range. • *Unstable or critically ill patients:* Daily if unstable, otherwise 2–3 times/wk. • *Stable hospitalized patients:* 1–2 times/wk.
TG	• *Baseline and initiation:* Baseline for PN; as medically indicated for EN. • *Unstable or critically ill patients:* Weekly for PN. More frequently if elevated >400 mg/dL. As medically indicated for EN. • *Stable hospitalized patients:* Weekly for PN; as medically indicated for EN.
CBC with differential[b]	• *Baseline and initiation:* Baseline for PN; as medically indicated for EN. • *Unstable or critically ill patients:* Weekly for PN; as medically indicated for EN. • *Stable hospitalized patients:* Weekly for PN; as medically indicated for EN.
AST, ALT, ALP, total bilirubin	• *Baseline and initiation:* Baseline for PN; as medically indicated for EN. • *Unstable or critically ill patients:* 1–3 times/wk for PN; as medically indicated for EN. • *Stable hospitalized patients:* Weekly to monthly for PN; as medically indicated for EN.

(continued)

Table 6.55 **Acute Enteral Nutrition or Parenteral Nutrition: Laboratory Tests and Frequency of Monitoring** (continued)

PT, INR	• *Baseline and initiation:* Baseline for PN; as medically indicated for EN.
	• *Unstable or critically ill patients:* Weekly for PN; as medically indicated for EN.
	• *Stable hospitalized patients:* Weekly for PN; as medically indicated for EN.

Abbreviations: EN, enteral nutrition; PN, parenteral nutrition; BUN, blood urea nitrogen; TG, triglycerides; CBC, complete blood count; AST, aspartate aminotransferase; ALT, alanine aminotransferase; ALP, alkaline phosphatase; PT, prothrombin time; INR, international normalized ratio; RBC, red blood cell; MCV, mean corpuscular volume; MCH, mean corpuscular hemoglobin; MCHC, mean corpuscular hemoglobin concentration; RDW, red cell distribution width.

[a]Listed for both EN and PN unless specified otherwise. Additional laboratory monitoring should be individualized, based on medical condition, route, tolerance to nutrition therapy, and previous laboratory value abnormalities.

[b]CBC with differential includes: white blood cell counts (neutrophils, lymphocytes, monocytes, eosinophils, and basophils), RBC count, hemoglobin concentration, hematocrit, platelet count, MCV, MCH, MCHC, and RDW.

Source: Data are from references 47 and 48.

Monitoring of Home Enteral Nutrition

Table 6.56 describes the frequency of monitoring required for selected laboratory tests used in home-based patients receiving EN (49–51).

Table 6.56 Home Enteral Nutrition: Laboratory Tests and Frequency of Monitoring

Laboratory Tests	Frequency of Monitoring
Sodium, potassium, chloride, glucose, BUN, creatinine, calcium, phosphorus, magnesium	• Obtain baseline, then monitor until abnormalities are corrected and stable. • The frequency of subsequent monitoring is based on severity of illness and is often done at routine physician visits as medically necessary based on diagnosis and during periods of EN intolerance. • If stable on EN, may only need to check laboratory results annually.
Albumin, CBC	• Baseline, then as medically indicated.

Abbreviations: BUN, blood urea nitrogen; EN, enteral nutrition; CBC, complete blood count.
Source: Data are from references 49, 50, and 51.

Monitoring of Home Parenteral Nutrition

To evaluate tolerance and effectiveness of HPN therapy and to help minimize complications, monitor laboratory tests at regular intervals and when the clinical condition changes. Daily patient record keeping should provide information on weight, intake/output records, temperature, and urinary or blood glucose, which can alert the clinician to order additional laboratory tests to evaluate hydration status, infection, and/or glucose control.

Although there are no national standards or evidence-based recommendations for routine laboratory monitoring of HPN patients, Table 6.57 provides general guidelines (52–56). Table 6.58 summarizes monitoring of metabolic bone disease, which should be done for patients on long-term HPN (53,55). Additional testing should be individualized, based on the medical condition, abnormal test results, and to assess effectiveness of changes to PN formula.

**Table 6.57   Home Parenteral Nutrition: Laboratory Tests and
Frequency of Monitoring[a]**

Laboratory Tests	Frequency of Monitoring
Sodium, potassium, chloride, bicarbonate, glucose, BUN, creatinine, calcium, phosphorus, magnesium	• Baseline, then weekly until stable, followed by monthly. • Frequency may taper to quarterly (every 3 mo) for stable, long-term patients.
Albumin, CBC, PT/INR	• Baseline, then monthly. • Frequency may taper to quarterly unless medical condition warrants more frequent monitoring.
Triglyceride	• Baseline, then as medically indicated if elevated or patient is at risk of hypertriglyceridemia (eg, poorly controlled diabetes, chronic renal failure, nephrotic syndrome, hypothyroidism, pancreatitis, or familial hypertriglyceridemia).
AST, ALT, ALP, GGT, total bilirubin	• Baseline, then weekly for 1–2 wk followed by monthly for 3 mo. • Frequency may taper to every 3 mo. • ALT and AST may rise within 1-3 wk after initiation of PN and can be associated with hepatic steatosis. • ALP and GGT may also rise (usually later) and may be associated with cholestasis. • An elevation in total bilirubin occurs less frequently and is typically observed last.
Vitamins, minerals, trace elements	• Optional baseline levels depending on underlying disease. • Every 6 mo to annually and if clinical suspicion of deficiency or toxicity (eg, vitamins B-12, folate, 25-OH vitamin D, A, E, and C; zinc, copper, selenium, manganese, and chromium).

(continued)

Table 6.57   Home Parenteral Nutrition: Laboratory Tests and Frequency of Monitoring^a (continued)

Laboratory Tests	Frequency of Monitoring
Iron studies (iron and ferritin)	• Optional baseline levels. • Every 3–6 mo if below normal or if treating for iron-deficiency anemia.
Triene:tetraene ratio	• Annually in patients at risk of EFAD (eg, those on lipid-free or low-lipid PN, severely malnourished, or those with physical signs/symptoms of EFAD).

Abbreviations: BUN, blood urea nitrogen; CBC, complete blood count; PT, prothrombin time; INR, international normalized ratio; ALT, alanine amino-transferase; AST, aspartate aminotransferase; PN, parenteral nutrition; ALP, alkaline phosphatase; GGT, gamma-glutamyl transferase; EFAD, essential fatty acid deficiency; HPN, home parenteral nutrition.

^aPatients discharged home on PN should be stable enough to require only weekly laboratory monitoring. Patients who have HPN started at home will initially require more frequent laboratory monitoring.

Source: Data are from references 52–56.

Table 6.58   Metabolic Bone Disease Monitoring in Patients Receiving Long-Term Home Parenteral Nutrition

- Evaluate bone mineral density using DXA every 1 to 2 y.
- Monitor serum calcium, phosphorus, and magnesium to maintain normal serum concentrations.
- Obtain a 24-hour urine collection for calcium and magnesium every 6 to 12 mo.
- Monitor baseline serum 25-hydroxy vitamin D and intact PTH annually or as needed.

Abbreviations: DXA, dual-energy X-ray absorptiometry; PTH, parathyroid hormone.

Source: Data are from references 53 and 55.

REFERENCES

1. Charney P. Nutrition assessment in the intensive care unit: Pre-albumin, C-reactive protein, or none of the above? *Support Line.* 2007;29:13–18.

2. Fuhrman MP, Charney P, Mueller CM. Hepatic proteins and nu-trition assessment. *J Am Diet Assoc*; 2004;104:1258–1264.

3. Russell MK. Laboratory monitoring. In: Matarese LE, Gottschlich MM, eds. *Contemporary Nutrition Support Practice: A Clinical Guide.* 2nd ed. St. Louis, MO: WB Saunders; 2003:45–62.

4. Vincent JL, Dubois MJ, Navickis RJ, Wilkes MM. Hypoalbuminemia in acute illness: Is there a rationale for intervention? A meta-analysis of cohort studies and controlled trials. *Ann Surg.* 2003;237:319–334.

5. Russell MK, Mueller C. Nutrition screening and assessment. In: Gottschlich MM, ed. *The A.S.P.E.N. Nutrition Support Core Curriculum: A Case-Based Approach—The Adult Patient.* Silver Spring, MD: ASPEN Publishers; 2007:163–186.

6. American Diabetes Association. Standards of medical care in diabetes—2015. *Diabetes Care.* 2015;38(Suppl 1):S1–S93. http://professional.diabetes.org/admin/UserFiles/0%20-%20 Sean/Documents/January%20Supplement%20Combined _Final.pdf. Accessed April 16, 2015.

7. Handelsman Y, Bloomgarden ZT, Grunberger G, Umpierrez G, Zimmerman RS, Bailey TS, Blonde L, Bray GA, Cohen AJ, Dagogo-Jack S, Davidson JA, Einhorn D, Ganda OP, Garber AJ, Garvey WT, Henry RR, Hirsch IB, Horton ES, Hurley DL, Jellinger PS, Jovanovič L, Lebovitz HE, LeRoith D, Levy P, McGill JB, Mechanick JI, Mestman JH, Moghissi ES, Orzeck EA, Pessah-Pollack R, Rosenblit PD, Vinik AI, Wyne K, Zangeneh F. American Association of Clinical Endocrinologists and American College of Endocrinology—Clinical practice guidelines for developing a diabetes mellitus comprehensive care plan—2015. *Endocr Pract.* 2015;21(Suppl 1):S1–S53.

8. Nasraway SA. Hyperglycemia during critical illness. *JPEN J Parenter Enteral Nutr.* 2006;30:254–258.

9. Van den Berghe G, Wouters P, Weekers F, Verwaest C, Bruyninckx F, Schetz M, Vlasselaers D, Ferdinande P, Lauwers P, Bouillon R. Intensive insulin therapy in the critically ill patients. *N Engl J Med.* 2001;345:1359–1367.

10. Van den Berghe G, Wilmer A, Hermans G, Meersseman W, Wouters PJ, Milants I, Van Wijngaerden E, Bobbaers H, Bouillon R. Intensive insulin therapy in the medical ICU. *N Engl J Med.* 2006;354:449–461.

11. Griesdale DE, de Souza RJ, van Dam RM, Heyland DK, Cook DJ, Malhotra A, Dhaliwal R, Henderson WR, Chittock DR, Finfer S, Talmor D. Intensive insulin therapy and mortality among critically ill patients: A meta-analysis including NICE-SUGAR study data. *CMAJ.* 2009;180:821–827.

12. Moghissi ES, Korytkowski MT, DiNardo M, Einhorn D, Hellman R, Hirsch IB, Inzucchi SE, Ismail-Beigi F, Kirkman MS, Umpierrez GE. American Association of Clinical Endocrinologists; American Diabetes Association. American Association of Clinical Endocrinologists and American Diabetes Association consensus statement on inpatient glycemic control. *Diabetes Care*. 2009;32(6):1119–1131.

13. Buse JB, Ginsberg HN, Bakris GL, Clark NG, Costa F, Eckel R, Fonseca V, Gerstein HC, Grundy S, Nesto RW, Pignone MP, Plutzky J, Porte D, Redberg R, Stitzel KF, Stone NJ. Primary prevention of cardiovascular diseases in people with diabetes mellitus: a scientific statement from the American Heart Association and the American Diabetes Association. *Diabetes Care*. 2007; 30:162–172.

14. Nathan DM, Cleary PA, Backlund JY, Genuth SM, Lachin JM, Orchard TJ, Raskin P, Zinman B. Intensive diabetes treatment and cardiovascular disease in patients with type 1 diabetes. *N Engl J Med*. 2005;353:2643–2653.

15. Pagana KD, Pagana TJ. *Mosby's Diagnostic and Laboratory Test Reference*. 10th ed. St. Louis, MO: Mosby; 2011.

16. Kee JL, ed. *Laboratory and Diagnostic Tests with Nursing Implications*. 7th ed. Upper Saddle River, NJ: Pearson Prentice Hall; 2005.

17. American Diabetes Association. Position statement. Hyperglycemic crises in diabetes. *Diabetes Care*. 2004;27(Suppl 1): S92–S102.

18. Heusel JW, Siggaard-Andersen O, Scott MG. Physiology and disorders of water, electrolyte, and acid-base metabolism. In: Burtis CA, Ashwood ER, eds. *Tietz Fundamentals of Clinical Chemistry*. 5th ed. Philadelphia, PA: WB Saunders; 2001:723–745.

19. Narins RG, Jones ER, Stom MC, Rudnick MR, Bastl CP. Diagnostic strategies in disorders of fluid, electrolyte and acid-base homeostasis. *Am J Med*. 1982;72:496–520.

20. Singer GG, Brenner BM. Fluid and electrolyte disturbances. In: Kasper DL, Fauci AS, Longo DL, Braunwald E, Hauser SL, Jameson JL, Loscalzo J, eds. *Harrison's Principles of Internal Medicine*. 17th ed. New York, NY: McGraw-Hill; 2005:252–263.

21. Whitmire SJ. Fluids, electrolytes and acid-base balance. In: Matarese LE, Gottschlich MM, eds. *Contemporary Nutrition Support Practice: A Clinical Guide*. 2nd ed. Philadelphia, PA: WB Saunders; 2003:127–144.

22. Avner ED. Clinical disorders of water metabolism: Hyponatremia and hypernatremia. *Pediatr Ann.* 1995;24:23–30.

23. Dickerson RN, Alexander KH, Minard G, Croce MA, Brown RO. Accuracy of methods to estimate ionized and "corrected" serum calcium concentrations in critically ill multiple trauma patients receiving specialized nutrition support. *JPEN J Parenter Enteral Nutr.* 2004;28:133–41.

24. Simmons JF, Assell CC. Acid-base basics. *Support Line.* 2001;23:6–11.

25. Boosalis MG. Micronutrients. In: Gottschlich MM, Fuhrman MP, Hammond KA, Holcombe BJ, Seidner DL, eds. *The Science and Practice of Nutrition Support: A Case-Based Core Curriculum.* Dubuque, IA: Kendall/Hunt; 2001:85–106.

26. Brittenham GM. Disorders of iron metabolism: Iron deficiency and overload. In: Hoffman R, Benz EJ, Shattil SJ, et al, eds. *Hematology: Basic Principles and Practice.* 3rd ed. New York, NY; 2000:397–418.

27. Klee GG. Cobalamin and folate evaluation: Measurement of methylmalonic acid and homocysteine vs vitamin B-12 and folate. *Clin Chem.* 2000;46:1277–1283.

28. Killip S, Bennet JM, Chambers MD. Iron deficiency anemia. *Am Fam Physician.* 2007;75:671–678.

29. DeBellis RJ. Anemia in critical care patients: Incidence, etiology, impact, management, and use of treatment guidelines and protocols. *Am J Health Syst Pharm.* 2007;64(3 Suppl 2):S14–S21.

30. McCormick DB, Klee GG. Vitamins. In: Burtis CA, Ashwood ER, eds. *Tietz Fundamentals of Clinical Chemistry.* 5th ed. Philadelphia, PA: WB Saunders; 2001:543–567.

31. Heimburger DC, McLaren DS, Shils ME. Clinical manifestations of human vitamin and mineral deficiencies and toxicities: A resume. In: Shils ME, Shike M, Ross AC, Caballero B, Cousins RJ, eds. *Modern Nutrition in Health and Disease.* 10th ed. Philadelphia, PA: Lippincott Williams & Wilkins; 2006:595–612.

32. Sauberlich HE: *Laboratory Tests for the Assessment of Nutritional Status.* 2nd ed. New York, NY: CRC Press; 1999.

33. Institute of Medicine. *Dietary Reference Intakes for Vitamin A, Vitamin K, Arsenic, Boron, Chromium, Copper, Iodine, Iron, Manganese, Molybdenum, Nickel, Silicon, Vanadium, and Zinc.* Washington, DC: National Academy Press; 2001.

34. Holick MF, Binkley NC, Bischoff-Ferrari HA, Gordon CM, Hanley DA, Heaney RP, Murad MH, Weaver CM. Evaluation, treatment and prevention of vitamin D deficiency: An Endocrine Society Clinical Guideline. *J Clin Endocrinol Metab* 2011;96:1911–1930.

35. McFarland LV. Meta-analysis of probiotics for the prevention of antibiotic associated diarrhea and the treatment of *Clostridium difficile* disease. *Am J Gastroenterol.* 2006;101:812–822.

36. Cohen SH, Gerding DN, Johnson S, Kelly CP, Loo VG, McDonald LC, Pepin J, Wilcox MH. Clinical practice guidelines for Clostridium difficile infection in adults: 2010 update by the Society for Healthcare Epidemiology of America (SHEA) and the Infectious Diseases Society of America (IDSA). *Infect Control Hosp Epidemiol.* 2010;31:431–455.

37. National Kidney Foundation. K/DOQI. Clinical practice guidelines: Nutrition in chronic renal failure. *Am J Kidney Dis.* 2000;35:(6 Suppl 2):S1–S140. www2.kidney.org/professionals /KDOQI/guidelines_nutrition/doqi_nut.html. Accessed May 7, 2015.

38. Bailie GR, Johnson CA, Mason NA, St. Peter WL, eds. Chronic Kidney Disease 2006: A Guide to Select NKF-KDOQI Guidelines and Recommendations. https://www.kidney.org/sites /default/files/docs/pharmacist_cpg.pdf. Accessed May 7, 2015.

39. National Kidney Foundation. K/DOQI clinical practice guidelines and clinical practice recommendations for anemia in chronic kidney disease. *Am J Kidney Dis.* 2006;47(Suppl 3): S1–S146. www2.kidney.org/professionals/KDOQI/guidelines _anemia. Accessed May 7, 2015.

40. McCray S, Walker S, Parrish CR. Much ado about refeeding. *Pract Gastroenterol.* 2005(Jan):26–41.

41. Bankhead R, Boullata J, Brantley S, Corkins M, Guenter P, Krenitsky J, Lyman B, Metheny NA, Mueller C, Robbins S, Wessel J. A.S.P.E.N. enteral nutrition practice recommendations. *JPEN J Parenter Enteral Nutr.* 2009;33:122–167.

42. Hise ME, Brown JC. Lipids. In: Gottschlich MM, ed. *The A.S.P.E.N. Nutrition Support Core Curriculum: A Case-Based Approach—the Adult Patient.* Silver Spring, MD: ASPEN Publishers; 2007:48–70.

43. Mayo Medical Laboratories. Reference values for fatty acid profile, essential, serum. www.mayomedicallaboratories.com /test-catalog/Clinical+and+Interpretive/82426. Accessed August 20, 2014.

44. Stone NJ, Robinson JG, Lichtenstein AH, Bairey Merz CN, Blum CB, Eckel RH, Goldberg AC, Gordon D, Levy D, Lloyd-Jones DM, McBride P, Schwartz JS, Shero ST, Smith SC Jr, Watson K, Wilson PWF. American College of Cardiology/American Heart Association Guideline on the treatment of blood cholesterol to reduce atherosclerotic cardiovascular risk in adults. *Circulation.* 2014;129(Suppl 2):S1–S29.

46. Alberti KG, Eckel RH, Grundy SM, Zimmet PZ, Cleeman JI, Donato KA, Fruchart JC, James WP, Loria CM, Smith SC Jr. Harmonizing the metabolic syndrome: A joint interim statement of the International Diabetes Federation Task Force on Epidemiology and Prevention; National Heart, Lung, and Blood Institute; American Heart Association; World Heart Federation; International Atherosclerosis Society; and International Association for the Study of Obesity. *Circulation.* 2009;120:1640–1645.

47. Mirtallo JM. Overview of parenteral nutrition. In: Gottschlich MM, ed. *The A.S.P.E.N. Nutrition Support Core Curriculum: A Case-Based Approach—The Adult Patient.* Silver Spring, MD: ASPEN Publishers; 2007.

48. Sacks GS, Mayhew S, Johnson D. Parental nutrition implementation and management. In: Merritt R, ed. *The A.S.P.E.N. Nutrition Support Practice Manual.* 2nd ed. Silver Spring, MD: ASPEN Publishers; 2005.

49. Ireton-Jones CS. Home enteral nutrition support in adults. In: Ireton-Jones CS, DeLegge MH, eds. *Handbook of Home Nutrition Support.* Sudbury, MA: Jones and Bartlett Publishers; 2007:83–101.

50. Pattinson A, Epp L. Home enteral nutrition. In: Charney P, Malone A. *Academy of Nutrition and Dietetics Pocket Guide to Enteral Nutrition.* 2nd ed. Chicago, IL: Academy of Nutrition and Dietetics; 2013:198–230.

51. Kovacevich DS, Orr ME. Considerations for home nutrition support. In: Merritt R, ed. *The A.S.P.E.N. Nutrition Support Practice Manual.* 2nd ed. Silver Spring, MD: ASPEN Publishers; 2005:371–377.

52. DeLegge MH, Ireton-Jones C. Home care. In: Gottschlich MM, ed. *The A.S.P.E.N. Nutrition Support Core Curriculum: A Case-Based Approach—the Adult Patient.* Silver Spring, MD: ASPEN Publishers; 2007:725–739.

53. Hamilton C, Seidner DL. Home parenteral nutrition in adults. In: Ireton-Jones CS, DeLegge MH, eds. *Handbook of Home Nutrition Support.* Sudbury, MA: Jones and Bartlett Publishers; 2007:115–152.

54. Hamilton C, Austin T. Home parenteral nutrition. In: Charney P, Malone A. *ADA Pocket Guide to Parenteral Nutrition.* Chicago, IL: American Dietetic Association; 2007:118–146.

55. Kelly DG. Guidelines and available products for parenteral vitamins and trace elements. *JPEN J Parenter Enteral Nutr.* 2002:26(5 Suppl):S34–S36.

56. Fuhrman MP. Micronutrient assessment in long-term home parenteral nutrition patients. *Nutr Clin Pract.* 2006;21:566–575.

Chapter 7

Client History

Mary J. Marian, DCN, RDN, CSO, FAND

INTRODUCTION

In the Nutrition Care Process Terminology (NCPT), the client history domain is comprised of (1):

- Personal history
- Patient/client/family medical/health history
- Social history

Using critical thinking and clinical reasoning skills, the registered dietitian nutritionist (RDN) assesses data from the client/patient history to determine whether a nutrition problem exists and what nutrition interventions and monitoring are necessary to resolve the nutrition problem or achieve established outcome goals via the Nutrition Care Process.

PERSONAL HISTORY

Personal history refers to the general patient/client information, including the person's age, sex/gender, race/ethnicity, and any physical disabilities or mobility issues (1).

Documentation of personal history can also note the patient's or client's language, literacy skills, education, and familial role. RDNs and other health care providers who take note of these factors can more effectively tailor their written and spoken communications to suit the individual patient/client, which may build trust/rapport in the patient-provider relationship, help elicit more insightful responses from the person being assessed, and improve compliance with the plan of care. Table 7.1 identifies selected resources on health literacy that may be of interest to RDNs.

Table 7.1   Health Literacy Resources

- Agency for Healthcare Research and Quality. Health Literacy Universal Precautions Toolkit. www.ahrq.gov/professionals /quality-patient-safety/quality-resources/tools/literacy-toolkit /index.html

- Centers for Disease Control and Prevention. Health Literacy. www.cdc.gov/healthliteracy

- Harvard School of Public Health. Health Literacy Studies. www.hsph.harvard.edu/healthliteracy

- Medline Plus. How to Write Easy-to-Read Health Materials. www.nlm.nih.gov/medlineplus/etr.html

- National Cancer Institute. Clear and Simple. www.nlm.nih.gov/medlineplus/etr.html

PATIENT/CLIENT/FAMILY MEDICAL/HEALTH HISTORY

The client/patient past medical history (PMH) is a critical component of nutrition assessment because this information often explains current findings or behaviors. The PMH also assists the RDN in determining appropriate nutrition interventions and guides selection of goals or outcomes for monitoring progress.

Items included in the PMH include past personal and family health history and risk/presence of chronic health conditions that may be related to nutrition and lifestyle.

In acute and ambulatory care, retrieval of historical information often begins with a thorough review of the medical record. Following review of the medical record, the RDN must corroborate information obtained from the record with patient/client or caregiver recall.

When the medical record is not available, the RDN must rely on information obtained from the patient/client or caregivers.

When patients/clients are referred from other health care providers, the RDN should contact the referring provider to clarify questions or concerns about the patient/client's PMH.

While each RDN will develop their own technique and style, every PMH must address common basic issues, including the following:

- Previous health conditions, including chronic conditions as well as previous acute health concerns that may be related to the current situation
- Past surgical history and surgical outcomes
- Medication history including prescribed and over-the-counter medications
- Prior use of alternative therapies
- Outcomes associated with previous treatments, medications or therapies
- Patient/client or caregiver perceptions related to previous treatment success or failure

Competency in assessing the PMH is enhanced with practice. More experienced RDNs will know when to ask for more information to clarify confusing or contradictory responses and when to shift questioning to better elucidate information that will inform the diagnostic process.

Table 7.2 includes the components of a detailed nutrition-oriented PMH (1,2).

Table 7.2   Components of the Past Medical History

Chief complaint
- Reason for seeking health care (diagnosis)
- Includes location, timing of onset and duration of symptoms
- Severity of symptoms
- Exacerbating/relieving factors; associated symptoms

Current health status
- Systematic review of patient's description of overall health:
  - Changes to hair, head, eyes, ears, nose, or throat
  - Concerns about skin and/or nails
  - Pressure ulcer(s): presence, stage(s), location
  - Symptoms associated with overhydration or underhydration
  - Cardiac/respiratory/abdominal status
  - Gynecological issues (eg, menopausal status, parity)
  - Musculoskeletal issues (eg, muscle pain, changes in functional status)
  - Concerns with immune function (eg, AIDS/HIV, severe infection)
  - Lifestyle history: nutrition, physical activity, tobacco/alcohol use, recreational drug use, occupational issues

Nutrition-related patient history
- Stated weight history (actual weight is considered part of the physical examination findings, not the patient history)
  - Compare stated weight and weight history to actual weight measurements from medical record
  - Note recent change in weight (timing and amount, gain or loss)
- Patient reports of factors influencing oral intake (eg, anorexia, chewing or swallowing difficulties, nausea, vomiting, diarrhea, constipation, steatorrhea, heartburn, gastroesophageal reflux, and/or abdominal pain)

Past medical/surgical history and chronic health conditions
Information-gathering shifts from current issues to issues that have been of concern in previous years.
- Past history of:
  - Alcoholism
  - Carcinoma
  - Cardiovascular disease (eg, hyperlipidemia, hypertension)
  - Respiratory disease(s) (eg, COPD, asthma, cystic fibrosis)

(continued)

Table 7.2 Components of the Past Medical History (continued)

- ◦ Developmental delay/cognition impaired
- ◦ Endocrine disorders (eg, diabetes, thyroid)
- ◦ Immune system disorders (eg, HIV/AIDS)
- ◦ Gastrointestinal issues (eg, esophageal/gastric reflux, gastroparesis, bariatric surgery, intestinal resections, inflammatory bowel disease, celiac disease, diverticulosis, irritable bowel syndrome, nausea, alterations in GI function, nutrient malabsorption, pancreatic insufficiency)
- ◦ Hepatic/accessory organ disease(s) (eg, pancreatic, gallbladder disorders)
- ◦ Hematological disorders (eg, anemia)
- ◦ Malnutrition
- ◦ Musculoskeletal disorders
- ◦ Neurological disorders (eg, Alzheimer disease, multiple sclerosis)
- ◦ Open wounds, draining fistulas/abscesses
- ◦ Renal disease

Psychiatric history
- Depression
- Eating disorders
- Psychosis

Surgical history
- History of operations; any complications noted (eg, infectious complications, fistula)
- GI tract resection or reconstruction
- Limb amputations that restrict mobility or independence (adjust anthropometrics as needed)
- Organ transplantation
- Paralysis
- Presence of enterocutaneous fistulas, ostomies, or poor wound healing

Diagnostic procedures
- Any for which prolonged NPO status is required

Medical therapies
- Chemotherapy or radiation therapy
- Dialysis
- Mechanical ventilation
- Ostomy
- Physical/speech/rehabilitation therapies

(continued)

Table 7.2   Components of the Past Medical History (continued)

Family health history
- Allergies (including food allergies)
- Cancer
- Cardiovascular disease
- Diabetes
- Food intolerances
- Genetic disorders that may affect nutritional status
- Gastrointestinal disorders
- Neuroendocrine disorders
- Obesity
- Osteoporosis

Oral health history
- Oral cavity health: gums, mucous membranes, lips, teeth, tongue
- Difficulty chewing and swallowing
- If patient uses dentures, question patient about ability to consume oral nutrition

Medications and dietary supplements
- Current/recent prescriptions (eg, anticonvulsants, immunosuppressants, insulin, steroids) and over-the-counter medications
- Drug-food and drug-nutrient interactions
- Dietary and botanical supplement use (eg, vitamins/minerals, fish oils, garlic, resveratrol)
- Complementary/alternative medicines
- Adverse effects that affect nutrient intake, nutrient absorption, excretion, and/or use

Source: Adapted from Cresci GA. Patient history. In: Charney P, Malone AM, eds. *ADA Pocket Guide to Nutrition Assessment.* 2nd ed. Chicago, IL: American Dietetic Association; 2009.

Surgical History

Tables 7.3 and 7.4 list potential adverse nutrition-related complications that may arise due to surgeries of the upper and lower gastrointestinal intestinal tract (2–4).

Table 7.3   **Potential Nutritional Consequences of Upper Gastrointestinal Surgery**[a]

Resection/replacement of esophagus
- Weight loss due to inadequate intake
- Early satiety with gastric pull-up procedures

Gastric pull-up
- Nausea/regurgitation due to loss of gastro/esophageal sphincter
- Increased protein loss due to catabolism
- Early satiety due to reduced reservoir capacity
- Rapid emptying of hypertonic fluids

Colonic interposition
- May require enteral/parenteral nutrition until oral intake is adequate
- Antidumping diet; patient may malabsorb fat/fat-soluble vitamins, simple sugars, and various vitamins/minerals
- Early satiety due to reduced reservoir capacity

Subtotal gastrectomy/vagotomy
- Early satiety due to reduced reservoir capacity
- Delayed gastric emptying of solids due to stasis
- Rapid emptying of hypertonic fluids
- Achlorhydria may result in difficulty tolerating fibrous foods and malabsorption of vitamins and minerals (eg, calcium, vitamins B-12 and D, iron)

Total gastrectomy
- Weight loss due to dumping syndrome/malabsorption, early satiety, anorexia, or inadequate intake
- Steatorrhea due to inadequate bile acids and pancreatic enzymes mixing with foods because of anastomotic changes
- Achlorhydria may result in difficulty tolerating fibrous foods and malabsorption of vitamins and minerals (eg, vitamin B-12, iron)
- Malabsorption may lead to anemia, metabolic bone disease, protein-energy malnutrition
- Bezoar formation
- Vitamin B-12 deficiency due to lack of intrinsic factor
- Lactose intolerance

(continued)

Table 7.3   Potential Nutritional Consequences of Upper Gastrointestinal Surgery[a] (continued)

Bariatric surgery
(Vertical gastric banding, adjustable gastric banding, Roux-en-Y gastric bypass, gastric sleeve)
- Protein-energy malnutrition from malabsorption related to dumping syndrome or inadequate bile acids and pancreatic enzymes mixing with foods because of anastomotic changes
- Dehydration and electrolyte abnormalities due to vomiting
- Malabsorption of vitamins/minerals due to achlorhydria (vitamin B-12, iron, calcium); decreased absorptive surface and/or bypassed site of absorption (iron, vitamin B-12, folate, thiamin, calcium); *or* decreased food intake
- Bezoar formation

Pancreaticoduodenectomy (Whipple procedure)
- Weight loss due to dumping syndrome, gastric stasis, nausea/vomiting, diabetes, and malabsorption due to resection of the pancreas

[a]Note that consequences may occur only with extensive disease process and resection.
Source: Adapted from Cresci GA. Patient history. In: Charney P, Malone AM, eds. *ADA Pocket Guide to Nutrition Assessment.* 2nd ed. Chicago, IL: American Dietetic Association; 2009.

Table 7.4   Potential Nutritional Consequences of Lower Gastrointestinal Surgery[a]

Proximal small bowel
- Malabsorption of vitamins/minerals (eg, calcium, magnesium, iron, vitamins A and D, folic acid)

Distal small bowel
- Protein-energy malnutrition due to malabsorption
- Fat malabsorption
- Malabsorption of fat-soluble vitamins (A, D, E, K)
- Bacterial overgrowth, especially if ileocecal valve is resected

(continued)

**Table 7.4   Potential Nutritional Consequences of Lower
Gastrointestinal Surgery[a] (continued)**

Colon
- Fluid and electrolyte (potassium, sodium, chloride)
  malabsorption
- Decreased production of short-chain fatty acids

---

[a]Note that consequences may occur only with extensive disease process and
resection.
Source: Adapted from Cresci GA. Patient history. In: Charney P, Malone
AM, eds. *ADA Pocket Guide to Nutrition Assessment.* 2nd ed. Chicago, IL:
American Dietetic Association; 2009.

Medication History

Table 7.5 identifies potential drug-nutrient interactions
that may require nutrition-related medication management and education (2,5,6). Table 7.6 lists potential drug-
induced nutritional and metabolic alterations (2).

**Table 7.5   Potential Drug-Nutrient Interactions That May
Require Nutrition-Related Medication Management
and Education[a]**

Amiodarone
- Grapefruit juice and dietary supplements that contain grapefruit
  bioflavonoids increase bioavailability of these medications
  because of inhibition of hepatic P-450 metabolism. Tangelos
  and Seville oranges may have a similar effect.

**Angiotensin-converting enzyme (ACE) inhibitors (benazepril,
enalapril, fosinopril, lisinopril, moexipril, perindorpil,
quinapril, ramipril, trandolapril)**
- Drugs increase serum potassium.
- Drugs deplete zinc.

Antianxiety/sedative hypnotics (buspirone, diazepam)
- Grapefruit juice and dietary supplements that contain grapefruit
  bioflavonoids increase bioavailability of these medications
  because of inhibition of hepatic P-450 metabolism. Tangelos
  and Seville oranges may have a similar effect.

(continued)

Table 7.5   Potential Drug-Nutrient Interactions That May Require Nutrition-Related Medication Management and Education[a] (continued)

Anticoagulants and platelet-aggregation inhibitors (cilostazol, warfarin)
- Grapefruit juice and dietary supplements that contain grapefruit bioflavonoids increase bioavailability of these medications because of inhibition of hepatic P-450 metabolism. Tangelos and Seville oranges may have a similar effect.
- Vitamin K decreases warfarin's effectiveness.
- Foods that make the urine acidic may decrease warfarin excretion.
- Foods that make the urine basic may increase warfarin excretion.

Antidepressants (clomipramine, sertraline)
- Grapefruit juice and dietary supplements that contain grapefruit bioflavonoids increase bioavailability of these medications because of inhibition of hepatic P-450 metabolism. Tangelos and Seville oranges may have a similar effect.

Benzodiazepines (eg, triazolam)
- Grapefruit juice and dietary supplements that contain grapefruit bioflavonoids increase bioavailability of these medications because of inhibition of hepatic P-450 metabolism. Tangelos and Seville oranges may have a similar effect.

Bile acid sequestrants (cholestryamine, colesevelam, colestipol)
- Drugs can possibly deplete vitamins A, B-12, D, E, K; folic acid; carotenoids; calcium, magnesium, iron, and zinc.

Calcium-channel blockers (amlodipine, felodipine, isradipine, nifedipine, nimodipine, nisoldipine, nitrendipine, verapamil)
- Grapefruit juice and dietary supplements that contain grapefruit bioflavonoids increase bioavailability of these medications because of inhibition of hepatic P-450 metabolism. Tangelos and Seville oranges may have a similar effect.

Carbamazepine
- Grapefruit juice and dietary supplements that contain grapefruit bioflavonoids increase bioavailability of these medications because of inhibition of hepatic P-450 metabolism. Tangelos and Seville oranges may have a similar effect.

(continued)

**Table 7.5   Potential Drug-Nutrient Interactions That May
Require Nutrition-Related Medication Management
and Education[a]** (continued)

Fibric acid derivatives (clofibrate, fenofibrate, gemfibrozil)
- Clofibrate and fenofibrate can lead to depletion of copper, vitamins B-12 and E, and zinc.
- Gemfibrozil depletes vitamin E and coenzyme Q10.

Fluoroquinolones (ciprofloxacin, levofloxacin)
- There is complexation of drug with divalent and trivalent cations in enteral feedings.
- Do not administer suspension drug with feeding tubes because of potential occlusion.
- For continuous enteral feedings, stop infusion for 2 hours before and 2 hours after drug if dose is administered via the GI tract.

Griseofulvin
- Take microsize forms of drug with or after a high-fat meal or whole milk to increase absorption.

HMG CoA–reductase inhibitors (atorvastatin, fluvastatin, lovastatin, pravastatin, rosuvastatin, simvastatin)
- Drugs may lead to depletion of coenzyme Q10 and vitamin E.
- Grapefruit juice and dietary supplements that contain grapefruit bioflavonoids increase bioavailability of these medications because of inhibition of hepatic P-450 metabolism. Tangelos and Seville oranges may have a similar effect.

Immunosuppressants (cyclosporine, sirolimus, tacrolimus)
- Grapefruit juice and dietary supplements that contain grapefruit bioflavonoids increase bioavailability of these medications because of inhibition of hepatic P-450 metabolism. Tangelos and Seville oranges may have a similar effect.

Levodopa
- Dietary amino acids compete with drug for absorptive sites, decreasing its bioavailability.

Levothyroxine
- Drug may bind to enteral feeding tubes, decreasing drug absorption.
- For continuous enteral feedings, stop infusion for 1 hour before and 2 hours after drug dose if it is administered via the GI tract.

(continued)

Table 7.5   **Potential Drug-Nutrient Interactions That May Require Nutrition-Related Medication Management and Education[a]** (continued)

Lipid-based medications (propofol)
- Drugs are based in 10% lipid emulsion, which may potentially increase total energy intake.

Loop diuretics (lasix, bumex)
- Drugs deplete potassium, magnesium, calcium, zinc, pyroxidene, thiamin, and ascorbic acid levels.

Metformin
- Drug can lead to depletion of vitamin B-12, folic acid, and coenzyme Q10.

Methadone
- Grapefruit juice and dietary supplements that contain grapefruit bioflavonoids increase bioavailability of these medications because of inhibition of hepatic P-450 metabolism. Tangelos and Seville oranges may have a similar effect.

Methotrexate
- Drug depletes folic acid.

Monoamine oxidase inhibitors (MAOIs)
- Patients on MAOIs should avoid foods high in tyramine and other pressor amines to prevent hypertensive crisis.

Phenytoin
- Enteral feedings decrease drug absorption.
- Hold enteral feedings for 2 hours before and 2 hours after dose.

Prednisone/dexamethasone
- Long-term therapy may result in need for supplementation of protein, calcium, potassium, phosphorus, folate, and vitamins A, C, and D.

Protease inhibitors (indinavir, saquinavir)
- Grapefruit juice and dietary supplements that contain grapefruit bioflavonoids increase bioavailability of these medications because of inhibition of hepatic P-450 metabolism. Tangelos and Seville oranges may have a similar effect.

Quinidine gluconate
- Absorption of drug increases when stomach is empty; patient may take with food or milk to decrease GI irritation.
- High potassium intake may increase the drug's effects.

(continued)

**Table 7.5   Potential Drug-Nutrient Interactions That May
Require Nutrition-Related Medication Management
and Education[a] (continued)**

Sildenafil
- Grapefruit juice and dietary supplements that contain grapefruit bioflavonoids increase bioavailability of these medications because of inhibition of hepatic P-450 metabolism. Tangelos and Seville oranges may have a similar effect.

Tetracycline
- Taking drug with iron-rich, calcium-rich, zinc-rich, and magnesium-rich foods can impair its absorption (due to chelation).

Thiazide and thiazide-like diuretics (chlorthalidone, chloro-thiazide, hydrocholorothiazide)
- Drugs deplete magnesium, potassium, and zinc.
- Drugs reduce calcium excretion.

[a]The registered dietitian nutritionist should use clinical judgment regarding additional drug-nutrient interaction patient education.
Source: Adapted from Cresci GA. Patient history. In: Charney P, Malone AM, eds *ADA Pocket Guide to Nutrition Assessment.* 2nd ed. Chicago, IL: American Dietetic Association; 2009.

Table 7.6   Drug-Induced Nutritional and Metabolic Alterations

Appetite, decreased
- Amphetamines, antibiotics, anticonvulsants, antineoplastics, fluoxetine, levodopa, thiazides, weight loss products/appetite suppressants

Appetite, increased
- Androgens, antihistamines, benzodiazepines, insulin, megestrol, phenothiazines, steroids, sulfonylureas

Altered taste
- Captopril, metronidazole (Flagyl)—metallic taste
- Chemotherapeutic agents (carboplatin, cisplatin, etoposide, interferon alpha, teniposide)
- Disulfiram
- Sulfonylureas

Dry mouth
- Antihistamines, atropine-like drugs, diuretics, radiation therapy, tricyclic antidepressants

(continued)

Table 7.6   Drug-Induced Nutritional and Metabolic Alterations
(continued)

Nausea/emesis
- Antibiotics, chemotherapeutic agents, thiazides

Diarrhea
- Antibiotics, cathartics, chemotherapy, cholinergics, lactulose, neomycin, prokinetic agents
- Enteral delivery of magnesium-containing medications, potassium-containing medications, hyperosmolar medications, sorbitol-containing medications

Constipation
- Barbiturates, opiates (morphine, codeine), vecuronium

Hyperglycemia
- Chemotherapeutic agents (L-asparaginase, interferon, methotrexate), steroids, tacrolimus, theophylline

Hypoglycemia
- Insulin, oral hypoglycemic agents, pentamidine

Hyperlipidemia
- Clevidipine, propofol

Altered fat metabolism/absorption
- Aluminum-containing antacids, androgens, cholestyramine, cyclosporine, estrogen, progestin

Sodium alterations
- *Loss:* Diuretics, laxatives, probenecid
- *Excess:* Penicillin G sodium, excessive delivery of normal saline

Potassium alterations
- *Loss:* Amphotericin B, diuretics, laxatives, probenecid
- *Excess:* Spironolactone, tacrolimus, penicillin G potassium (reduced loss)

Phosphorus alterations
- *Loss:* Binders (aluminum, calcium, magnesium, sevelamer [renagel], sucralfate), corticosteroids, furosemide, thiazides
- *Excess:* Several doses of phosphorus-containing bowel preparation kits (eg, Fleets, Phospha-soda), especially for renal failure patients

(continued)

Table 7.6 Drug-Induced Nutritional and Metabolic Alterations
(continued)

Magnesium alterations
- *Loss*: Amphotericin B, carbenicillin, ciprofloxacin, cisplatin, cyclosporine, diuretics, pentamidine, probenecid, tacrolimus
- *Excess*: Bowel preparation (milk of magnesia)

Calcium loss
- Amphotericin B, calcitonin, cisplatin, corticosteroids, furosemide, mithramycin, probenecid, phenytoin, pentamidine, triamterene

Source: Adapted from Cresci GA. Patient history. In: Charney P, Malone AM, eds. *ADA Pocket Guide to Nutrition Assessment.* 2nd ed. Chicago, IL: American Dietetic Association; 2009.

SOCIAL HISTORY

A social history contains information regarding an individual's socioeconomic status, housing situation, access to a social support system, access to medical care, activity level, food purchasing and preparation capabilities, and religious practices. Understanding the social background allows the health care provider to tailor the nutrition care plan to better meet the patient's needs. Table 7.7 describes a detailed nutrition-oriented social history (2,7–9).

Table 7.7 Components of a Social History

Socioeconomic status
- Employment status
- Income from Social Security
- Government programs: Food stamps, Special Supplemental Nutrition Program for Women, Infants and Children (WIC), Medicare, Medicaid, others
- Available food storage: eg, type of refrigeration (full-sized vs small "dorm-sized" unit or ice chest)
- Food delivery programs, such as Meals on Wheels

(continued)

Table 7.7   Components of a Social History (continued)

Housing situation
- Lives alone
- Urban vs rural area
- Lives with family member or caregiver
- Lives in group home, skilled care facility, etc
- Incarceration (jail, prison)
- Homeless

Social and medical support
- Family members
- Friends
- Access to medical care (eg, Medicare, Medicaid, private medical insurance)

History of recent crisis
- Job loss
- Family member death
- Trauma, surgery
- Daily stress level

Activity level
- Exercise (sedentary, moderately active, very active)
- House- or bed-bound
- Ability to perform activities of daily living
- Tremors (eg, Parkinson's disease)
- Posturing
- Seizure activity

Meal preparation
- Who purchases and prepares foods? What is their ability and skill to prepare food?
- Meal preparation facilities (full kitchen vs "hot plate," microwave)
- Shopping facilities (grocery store vs convenience markets)
- Dining out

Other factors
- Religious and cultural dietary practices
- Use of tobacco products
- Alcohol and drug use or abuse
- Support group attendance (weight control, substance abuse, etc)
- Home nutrition support therapy or nursing care

Source: Adapted from Cresci GA. Patient history. In: Charney P, Malone AM, eds. *ADA Pocket Guide to Nutrition Assessment.* 2nd ed. Chicago, IL: American Dietetic Association; 2009.

REFERENCES

1. Academy of Nutrition and Dietetics. eNCPT: Nutrition Care Process Terminology. 2014. https://ncpt.webauthor.com. Accessed April 13, 2015.

2. Cresci GA. Patient history. In: *ADA Pocket Guide to Nutrition Assessment.* 2nd ed. Chicago, IL: American Dietetic Association; 2009:20–39.

3. Rees Parrish C, Krenitsky J, Willcutts K, Radigan AE. Gastrointestinal disease. In: Gottschlich M, DeLegge M, Mattox T, Mueller C, Worthington P, eds. *The A.S.P.E.N. Nutrition Support Core Curriculum: A Case-Based Approach—The Adult Patient.* Silver Spring, MD: ASPEN; 2007:508–539.

4. Cresci GA, Gottschlich MM, Mayes T, Mueller C. Trauma, surgery, and burns nutrition, In: Gottschlich M, DeLegge M, Mattox T, Mueller C, Worthington P, eds. *The A.S.P.E.N. Nutrition Support Core Curriculum: A Case-Based Approach—The Adult Patient.* Silver Spring, MD: ASPEN; 2007:455–476.

5. US National Library of Medicine. Medline Plus: Drugs, Supplements, and Herbal Information. www.nlm.nih.gov/medlineplus/druginformation.html. Accessed April 14, 2015.

6. Rollins C. Drug-nutrient interactions. In: Gottschlich M, DeLegge M, Mattox T, Mueller C, Worthington P, eds. *The A.S.P.E.N. Nutrition Support Core Curriculum: A Case-Based Approach—The Adult Patient.* Silver Spring, MD: ASPEN; 2007:340–359.

7. Russell MK, Mueller C. Nutrition screening and assessment. In: Gottschlich M, DeLegge M, Mattox T, Mueller C, Worthington P, eds. *The A.S.P.E.N. Nutrition Support Core Curriculum: A Case-Based Approach—The Adult Patient.* Silver Spring, MD: ASPEN; 2007:163–186.

8. Hammond K. History and physical examination. In: Matarese L, Gottschilch M, eds. *Contemporary Nutrition Support Practice: A Clinical Guide.* Philadelphia, PA: WB Saunders; 1998:17–32.

9. Hopkins B. Assessment of nutritional status. In: Gottschlich M, Matarese L, Shronts E, eds. *Nutrition Support Dietetics: Core Curriculum.* Silver Spring, MD: ASPEN; 1993:15–70.

Chapter 8

Nutrient Requirements

Ainsley Malone, MS, RD, LD, CNSC,
FAND, FASPEN and
Mary Krystofiak Russell, MS, RDN,
LDN, FAND

INTRODUCTION

This chapter addresses ways to measure, estimate, and interpret a patient's energy, protein, fluid, and micronutrient requirements. These requirements provide a point of comparison for assessing the patient's actual nutrient intake and inform the registered dietitian nutritionist's (RDN's) determination of the patient's nutrition diagnosis (or diagnoses) and the individualized nutrition prescription (1).

METHODS FOR DETERMINING ENERGY REQUIREMENTS

Energy requirements can be measured using indirect calorimetry or estimated using one of several predictive equations.

Indirect Calorimetry

Indirect calorimetry uses measurements of inspired and expired gas volumes to determine energy expenditure. Indirect calorimetry closely approximates actual energy

213

expenditure because it accounts for variability in energy expenditure caused by changes in metabolic state.

Predictive Equations

In 2006 and 2012, the Academy of Nutrition and Dietetics (Academy) completed systematic reviews of available predictive equations for determining energy requirements and clarified which methods are most closely aligned to actual energy expenditure as measured by indirect calorimetry (2,3). The Academy evidence analysis projects focus on the estimation of energy requirements for three patient populations:

- Noncritically ill patients
- Critically ill patients
- Patients who are obese (with a body mass index [BMI] ≥30)

Figure 8.1 outlines an algorithmic approach to estimating energy requirements in hospitalized patients. More detailed information about predictive equations for each population is presented in the subsequent sections of this chapter.

Figure 8.1   Using Predictive Equations to Estimate Energy Requirements

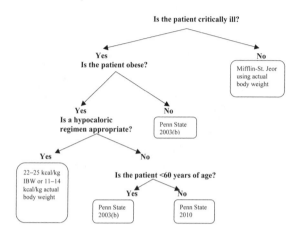

ENERGY REQUIREMENTS FOR NONCRITICALLY ILL PATIENTS

The Academy (2,3) has made the following recommendations for determining energy requirements in noncritically ill patients:

- If possible, resting metabolic rate (RMR) should be measured (eg, through use of indirect calorimetry).
- If RMR cannot be measured, the Mifflin-St. Jeor equation (see Table 8.1 [4]) using actual weight is the most accurate method for estimating RMR for overweight and obese individuals. *Strong, Conditional* (applies to those who meet the condition that RMR cannot be measured)

Table 8.1   Mifflin-St. Jeor Equations for Estimating Resting Metabolic Rate

Men

$$RMR = (9.99W) + (6.25H) - (4.92A) + 5$$

Women

$$RMR = (9.99W) + (6.25H) - (4.92A) - 161$$

Where: RMR = resting metabolic rate (energy expenditure) in kilocalories; W = actual weight in kilograms; H = height in centimeters; A = age in years.

Source: Data are from reference 4.

ENERGY REQUIREMENTS FOR CRITICALLY ILL PATIENTS

Indirect Calorimetry

According to the Academy's Critical Illness Evidence-Based Nutrition Practice Guideline (3), "indirect calorimetry is the standard for determination of RMR in critically ill patients." However, the following issues may limit the effective use of IC (5):

- Leaks may occur in the ventilator circuit, endotracheal tube cuffs, or uncuffed tubes, through chest tubes or bronchopleural fistula.
- Peritoneal and hemodialysis procedures remove carbon dioxide during the treatment, and acid-base levels require a few hours after the treatment to stabilize. Patients should not be measured during or for four hours after these dialysis treatments.
- Inaccurate measures may be caused by:
  - Instability of delivered oxygen concentration (fraction of inspired oxygen; FiO_2) within a breath or breath-to-breath, due to changes in source gas pressure and ventilator blender/mixing characteristics
  - FiO_2 greater than 60%

- Inability to separate inspired from expired gases, due to bias flow with intermittent mandatory ventilation systems
- Anesthetic gases other than oxygen, carbon dioxide, and nitrogen in the system
- Water vapor presence
- Inappropriate calibration
- Total circuit flow exceeding internal gas flow of calorimeter
- Leaks within the calorimeter
- Inadequate measurement length

See Table 8.2 for recommendations for improving accuracy of performing indirect calorimetry (6).

Table 8.2   Recommendations for Improving Accuracy of Indirect Calorimetry

- Patients have rested in a supine position (in bed or a recliner) for more than 30 minutes before the study to avoid the effects of voluntary activity on REE.
- Patients receiving intermittent feedings (i.e., bolus enteral feeding, cyclic enteral or parenteral nutrition, or meals) are studied approximately 1 hour after the feeding if thermogenesis is be included in the REE or 4 hours after the feeding if it is not.
- The rate and composition of nutrients being infused on a continuous basis are stable for at least 12 hours before and during the study.
- Measurements are made in a quiet, thermoneutral environment.
- All sources of supplemental oxygen (ie, nasal cannulas, masks, or tracheostomy collars) are turned off during routine room air measurements, if medically feasible.
- The fraction of inspired oxygen (FiO_2) remains constant during the measurement.
- The study is delayed for 90 minutes if changes are required in ventilatory settings.

(continued)

Table 8.2   Recommendations for Improving Accuracy of Indirect Calorimetry (continued)

- The patient has usual patterns of voluntary skeletal muscle activity (movement of the extremities) during the study.
- No leaks in the sampling system are present.
- All data used to derive REE and RQ are taken from a period of equilibrium or a steady state that has been identified according to statistically defined guidelines.
- The patient has not received general anesthesia within 6 to 8 hours before the study.
- If the patient is in pain or agitated, analgesics or sedatives should be given at least 30 minutes before the study when clinically possible; analgesics and sedatives administered will be documented, and this information will be considered during interpretation of the study.
- The study will be delayed 3 to 4 hours after hemodialysis.
- The study will be delayed 1 hour after painful procedures have been performed.
- Routine nursing care or activities involving other health care professionals should be avoided during the study.

Source: Reprinted from reference 6: Wooley JA, Sax, HC. Indirect calorimetry: Applications to practice. *Nutr Clin Pract.* 2003;18:434–439. Reprinted by permission of Sage Publications.

Respiratory Quotient

Respiratory quotient (RQ), a measure of carbon dioxide produced over oxygen consumed, has historically been used to evaluate substrate utilization (7). According to the Academy's Evidence Analysis Library (EAL) (8):

> If RQ is below 0.7 or above 1, then repeated measures are necessary under more optimal conditions. An RQ under 0.7 suggests hypoventilation (inadequate removal of metabolic carbon dioxide from the blood to the lung) or prolonged fasting. An RQ above 1, in the absence of overfeeding, suggests hyperventilation (removal of carbon dioxide from the blood to the lung in excess of the amount produced by metabolism) or inaccurate gas collection. *Strong, Conditional.*

Interpretation of RMR and RQ (9)

- The validity of the IC measurement needs to be assessed prior to its interpretation. Confirmation of a steady state during testing and an RQ within physiological range 0.67–1.3 verifies test validity.
- For continuous PN or EN feedings, no adjustment to the RMR is needed in prescribing energy intake
- For intermittent, bolus or cycle feedings, 5% of the RMR should be added in prescribing energy intake.
- RQ measurements can be falsely low due to:
  - Oxidation of ethanol and ketones
  - Diabetic ketoacidosis
  - Underfeeding
  - Inflammatory related substrate shifts
  - Hypoventilation
  - Technical difficulties
  - High rates of urinary glucose excretion
  - Lipolysis
- RQ measurements can be falsely high due to:
  - Excess carbon dioxide production
  - Provision of exogenous buffering agents such as sodium bicarbonate
  - Lipogenesis
  - Overfeeding

Predictive Equations

Table 8.3 lists the predictive equations recommended in the Academy's 2012 Critical Illness Evidence-Based Nutrition Practice Guideline to assess energy requirements in critically ill patients when indirect calorimetry is not available (3,10–12). Table 8.4 surveys the Academy's evidence analysis of the accuracy of multiple predictive equations that have been developed for use in critically ill patients (10).

Table 8.3 Recommended Equations for Estimating Energy Requirements in Mechanically Ventilated, Critically Ill Adults

Penn State University (2003b)[b]:

$$RMR = [(BMR \times 0.96) \times (V_E \times 31)] + (T_{max} \times 167) - 6,212$$

Recommended for:
- Nonobese patients
- Obese patients ages <60 y

Penn State University (2010)[b]:

$$RMR = [(BMR \times 0.71) \times (V_E \times 64)] + (T_{max} \times 85) - 3,085$$

Recommended for obese patients ages ≥60 y

[a]These recommendations are graded *Fair, Conditional* by the Academy of Nutrition and Dietetics.
[b]Where: BMR = basal metabolic rate (kcal/d) calculated by the Mifflin-St. Jeor equation (see Table 8.2); V_E = minute ventilation (L/min); T_{max} = maximum daily body temperature (degrees Celsius).
Source: Data are from references 3 and 10–12.

Table 8.4 Evaluation of Predictive Equations for RMR in Critically Ill Patients

Predictive Equation	Accuracy Rate (Over-estimation or Underestimation)
PSU 2003(b) for nonobese	Range: 70%–74% (Not reported)
PSU 2003(b) for obese, age <60 y	Mean: 70% (Not reported)
PSU 2003(b) for obese, age ≥60 years	Mean: 74% (Not reported)
HBE w/o adjustments	Range: 26%–35% (–1000 kcal)
HBE w/stress and activity factors	Range: 15%–51% (±900 kcal)
HBE w/weight adjustment for obesity	Mean: 55% (34% underprediction; 62% overprediction)

(continued)

**Table 8.4   Evaluation of Predictive Equations for RMR in
Critically Ill Patients** (continued)

Predictive Equation	Accuracy Rate (Over-estimation or Underestimation)
IJ 1992	Range: 28%–60% (Not reported)
IJ 1997	Range: 15%–48% (Not reported)
MSJ × 1.25	Mean: 50% (Not reported)
Swinamer	Range: 45%–61% (Biased toward overprediction)
Brandi	Mean: 61% (Not reported)
Faisy	Mean: 53% (Not reported)

Abbreviations: PSU, Penn State University; HBE, Harris-Benedict equation; IJ, Ireton-Jones; MSJ, Mifflin-St. Jeor.
Source: Data are from reference 10.

HYPOCALORIC HIGH-PROTEIN REGIMEN FOR OBESE PATIENTS (BMI ≥ 30)

According to the Academy's Evidence Analysis Library (13):

> In obese, critically ill adults, the registered dietitian/ nutritionists (RDN) may consider hypocaloric, high-protein feedings. Very limited research in patients primarily receiving enteral nutrition (EN) shows that the effect of hypocaloric, high-protein feeding (<20 kcal per kg adjusted body weight [ABW] and 2 g protein per kg ideal body weight [IBW]) promoted shorter intensive care unit (ICU) stays, although total hospital length of stay (LOS) did not differ. Nitrogen balance was not adversely affected. The effect of this feeding regimen on infectious complications, days on

mechanical ventilation, mortality and cost of care is unsubstantiated. *Weak, Conditional.*

Recommendations from the A.S.P.E.N./SCCM Guidelines for the provision and assessment of nutrition support therapy in the adult critically ill patient (14) support this approach and suggest using:

- 11–14 kcal/kg actual weight *or*
- 22–25 kcal/kg IBW (see Chapter 4 for more information about IBW)

Both acutely ill and critically ill obese patients have been studied using this caloric approach (15,16).

A.S.P.E.N.'s clinical guidelines on nutrition support for adult patients with obesity (17) suggest a trial of hypocaloric, high-protein feeding in patients who do not have severe renal or hepatic dysfunction. Hypocaloric feeding may be started with the following:

- 50%–70% of estimated energy needs *or*
- < 14 kcal/kg actual weight

PROTEIN REQUIREMENTS

Protein requirements are based on nutritional status, presence of disease or injury, and physiological capability to metabolize and utilize protein.

- Protein requirements can be determined through calculation of nitrogen balance, which compares nitrogen (protein) intake to nitrogen (protein) output. RDNs should note that there are limitations to use of nitrogen balance, including inaccurate urine collection and presence of renal dysfunction.

- For critically ill and/or metabolically stressed patients, current clinical practice guidelines recommend providing energy to meet metabolic demand, and, assuming adequate organ function, 1.5 g of protein/kg/d (range 1.2–2 g/kg/d) (14). Provision of protein in larger doses does not typically mitigate a negative nitrogen balance, although additional protein may be warranted in patients with large burns, multiple trauma, protein-losing enteropathies, necrotizing fasciitis and traumatic brain injuries (18–21).

- In the critically ill obese patient, high-protein feeding may be started with 1.2 g/kg actual weight or 2–2.5 g/kg IBW, with adjustment of goal protein intake by the results of nitrogen balance. Patients with hepatic and/or renal dysfunction may require less protein than critically ill patients with adequate organ function. For example, obese patients with renal dysfunction (serum creatinine >2 mg/dL) or hepatic dysfunction (serum total bilirubin >3 mg/dL) should be provided with moderate protein intake of 1.5 g/kg/ IBW (17).

- However, automatic protein restriction for patients with hepatic or renal dysfunction is not appropriate. Nutritional status, clinical condition, and use of renal replacement therapy will affect protein requirements (14,21–25). Close patient monitoring is essential if protein intake is restricted.

- Refer to Table 8.5 for a summary of protein requirements for adults (15,18,26–29).

Chapter 8

Table 8.5   Daily Protein Requirement for Adults

Condition Descriptor	Protein Requirement
DRI reference	0.8 g/kg
Adult maintenance	0.8–1 g/kg
Older adults	1 g/kg
Renal disease: predialysis	0.6–0.8 g/kg
Renal disease: hemodialysis	1.2–1.3 g/kg
Renal disease: peritoneal dialysis	>1.3 g/kg
Renal disease: CRRT	>1.5–2.5 g/kg
Hepatitis (acute or chronic)	1–1.5 g/kg
Liver disease/cirrhosis	1.2–1.6 g/kg
Cancer	1–1.5 g/kg
Cancer cachexia	1.5–2.5 g/kg
Bone marrow transplant	1.5 g/kg
Inflammatory bowel disease	1–1.5 g/kg
Short bowel syndrome	1.5–2 g/kg
BMI >27, normal renal and hepatic function	1.5–2 g/kg IBW (with hypocaloric feeding)
Obesity class I or II, trauma (ICU)	1.9 g/kg IBW (with hypocaloric feeding)
Obesity class III, trauma (ICU)	2.5 g/kg IBW (with hypocaloric feeding)
Solid organ transplant: acute posttransplant	1.5–2 g/kg
Solid organ transplant: long-term	1 g/kg
Pregnancy	+25 g/d
Pulmonary disease	1.2–1.5 g/kg
Critical illness (including burns, sepsis, and traumatic brain injury)	1.5–2 g/kg
Stroke	1–1.25 g/kg

Abbreviations: BMI, body mass index; CRRT, continuous renal replacement therapy; DRI, Dietary Reference Intake; IBW, ideal body weight; ICU, intensive care unit.
Source: Data are from references 15, 18, and 26–29.

FLUID AND ELECTROLYTE MANAGEMENT

The goals of fluid management include maintenance of adequate hydration, tissue perfusion, and electrolyte balance. Insensible losses, measured losses (stool, urine, wound and/or ostomy drainage) and alterations in fluid balance due to metabolic changes (fever and hyperthyroidism) or medical therapy (diuretics) must be considered. For more information on this topic, see references 30–36.

Laboratory and Clinical Assessment

No single laboratory test is diagnostic for volume status changes. Electrolyte abnormalities may be detected first by a laboratory test. (See Chapter 6 for additional information on laboratory testing.)

Clinical examination, understanding of the disease state or condition, laboratory monitoring and in some cases hemodynamic monitoring, are needed to appropriately assess and treat fluid and electrolyte abnormalities. In addition, knowledge of the composition of body fluids will enable the clinician to choose the appropriate replacement strategies for fluid and electrolyte derangements (see Tables 8.6–8.13) (20–23,33,35).

Table 8.6 **Volume and Electrolyte Composition of Selected Body Fluids**

Fluid	Electrolytes, mEq/L				Volume, L/d
	Na$^+$	K$^+$	Cl$^-$	HCO$_3^-$	
Saliva	10–30	20–30	10–35	15–30	1–1.5
Gastric, pH <4	60	10	90		2.5
Gastric, pH >4	100	10	100		2
Bile	145	5	100–110	35–40	1.5
Duodenal	140	5	80	50	
Pancreatic	140	5	75	90	0.7–1
Ileal	130–140	5–10	104–110	30	3–3.5
Cecal	80	20	50	20	
Colonic	60	30	40	20	0.5–2
Sweat	50	5	55		0–3
New ileostomy	130	20	110	30	0.5–2
Adapted ileostomy	50	5	30	25	0.4
Colostomy	50	10	40	20	0.3–2

Source: Reprinted from reference 35: Lyerly H, Gaynor J. *The Handbook of Surgical Intensive Care.* 3rd ed. St. Louis, MO: Mosby; 1992:410. Reprinted with permission from Elsevier.

Table 8.7   Electrolyte Concentrations and Osmolality of Common Intravenous Fluids

Intravenous Fluid	Sodium, mEq/L	Potassium, mEq/L	Calcium, mEq/L	Chloride, mEq/L	Lactate, mEq/L	Osmolality, mOsm/L
5% dextrose solution	0	0	0	0	0	278
10% dextrose solution	0	0	0	0	0	505
0.9% NaCl (normal saline) solution	154	0	0	154	0	308
Sodium lactate solution	167	0	0	0	167	334
5% dextrose, 0.45% NaCl (half normal saline) solution	77	0	0	77	0	406
5% dextrose, 0.9% NaCl (normal saline) solution	154	0	0	154	0	560
Ringer's solution	147.5	4	4.5	156	0	309
Lactated Ringer's solution	130	4	3	109	28	273
5% dextrose in Ringer's solution	147.5	4	4.5	156	0	561
5% dextrose in lactated Ringer's solution	130	4	3	109	28	525

Source: Reprinted with permission from reference 33: Whitmire, SJ. Fluid, electrolytes, and acid-base balance. In: Matarese L, Gottschlich M, eds. *Contemporary Nutrition Support Practice.* 2nd ed. Philadelphia, PA: WB Saunders; 2003:127. Copyright © Laura Matarese and Michelle Gottschlich.

Table 8.8   Factors That Affect Fluid Requirements

Factor	Increase in Fluid Requirement
Fever	12.5% for each 1°C above normal
Sweating	10%–25%
Hyperventilation	10%–60%
Hyperthyroidism	25%–50%
Extraordinary gastric and/or renal fluid losses	Varies (base adjustment on average 24-h output)

Source: Reprinted with permission from reference 33: Whitmire, SJ. Fluid, electrolytes, and acid-base balance. In: Matarese L, Gottschlich M, eds. *Contemporary Nutrition Support Practice.* Philadelphia, PA: WB Saunders; 1998:131. Copyright © Laura Matarese and Michelle Gottschlich.

Table 8.9   Magnesium Supplementation Guidelines

Magnesium sulfate = 8 mEq magnesium per g

Enteral route
- Up to 2 mEq/kg body weight if normal renal function for repletion
- 10 mL milk of magnesia or 600 mg Mg oxide = 20 mEq Mg
- Gastrointestinal tolerance can be a limiting factor.

Parenteral route
- 32–64 mEq magnesium sulfate, up to 1.5 mEq/kg, for severe hypomagnesemia (serum level < 1 mg/dL)
- 8–32 mEq magnesium sulfate, up to 1 mEq/kg, for mild to moderate hypomagnesemia (serum level 1–1.5 mg/dL)
- May require several days to correct
- Reduce doses by ~50% for persons with renal impairment.

Source: Data are from references 17–20.

Table 8.10   Phosphorus Supplementation Guidelines

- 1 mmol = 31 mg elemental phosphorus
- Potassium phosphate is preferred over sodium phosphate when serum potassium level < 4 mEq/L.

(continued)

Table 8.10   Phosphorus Supplementation Guidelines
(continued)

Enteral route
* Sodium phosphate 5 mL, 3 times per day (4.2 mmol phos/mL) or potassium phosphate (1.25 g: 8 mmol phos, 14.2 mEq K) for mild asymptomatic hypophosphatemia

Parenteral route
* 1 mmol/kg for severe hypophosphatemia (serum level <1.5 mg/dL)
* 0.64 mmol/kg >6 h for moderate hypophosphatemia (serum level 1.6–2.2 mg/dL)
* 0.32 mmol/kg >6 h for mild hypophosphatemia (serum level 2.3–3 mg/dL)
* Phosphorus administered at a rate not to exceed 7.5 mmol phosphorus/h
* Reduce doses by ~50% for persons with renal impairment.
* Recheck serum levels periodically.

Source: Data are from references 20–23.

Table 8.11   Potassium Supplementation Guidelines

* Review EKG for ventricular arrhythmias.
* Correct alkalosis.
* Correct concurrent hypomagnesemia.
* Continuous cardiac monitoring is recommended for infusion rates >10 mEq potassium per h.

Enteral route
* 80–120 mEq/d for repletion
* Each dose: 40 mEq via tube or orally
* Potassium supplements are best administered orally in a moderate dosage over a period of days to weeks to achieve full repletion.
* Gastrointestinal tolerance can be a limiting factor.

Parenteral route
* Do not exceed 10 mEq/h via peripheral, 40 mEq/h via central; usual IV infusion rate is 10–20 mEq/h
* Suggested repletion schedule:
  ○ Serum level 2.5–3.4 mg/dL: 20–40 mEq
  ○ Serum level <2.5 mg/dL: replace 40–80 mEq in divided doses
  ○ Reduce doses by ~50% for persons with renal impairment.

Source: Data are from references 20–23.

Table 8.12   Sodium Supplementation Guidelines

- Consider check of plasma osmolality and urinary sodium.
- Treatment depends on specific sodium alteration (see below).
- Do not correct > 50% of calculated Na deficiency in first 24 hours; correct 1 mEq/h

Parenteral route
- Hypovolemic hypotonic hyponatremia: isotonic saline
- Hypervolemic isotonic hyponatremia: fluid restriction, +/– diuresis
- Isovolemic hypotonic hyponatremia: fluid restriction, +/– diuresis
- Severe symptomatic hyponatremia: fluid restriction; 3% hypertonic NaCL until Na > 120 mg/dL

Source: Data are from references 20–23.

Table 8.13   Calculation of Fluid Deficit

$$\text{Body H}_2\text{0 deficit} = \text{Normal TBW} - \text{Current TBW}$$

$$\text{Normal TBW (L)} = \% \text{ TBW} \times \text{Normal body weight (kg)}$$

$$\text{Current TBW (L)} = \frac{\text{Normal serum Na}^+ \text{ (140 mEq/L)}}{\text{Measured serum Na}^+ \text{ (mEq/L)}} \times \text{Normal TBW (L)}$$

Alternatively, based on algebraic manipulation of the above equations:

$$\text{Calculated H}_2\text{0 deficit} = \% \text{ TBW} \times \text{Normal body weight (kg)}$$
$$\times \frac{1 - \text{Normal serum Na}^+ \text{ (140 mEq/L)}}{\text{Measured serum Na}^+ \text{ (mEq/L)}}$$

Source: Adapted with permission from reference 27: Matarese L, Gottschlich M, eds. *Contemporary Nutrition Support Practice.* Philadelphia, PA: WB Saunders; 1998:131. Copyright © Laura Matarese and Michelle Gottschlich.

Estimating Fluid Needs

Table 8.14 presents various methods for estimating fluid needs (33,36). The Academy of Nutrition and Dietetics evidence analysis project on hydration (2007) evaluated three of the methods (weight, RDA, and fluid balance) and concluded that "there was no evidence found to establish or validate the equations. These three equations have, however, been cited extensively in many well-respected documents and widely used in clinical practice. Well-designed studies are needed to determine and validate predictive equations to estimate fluid requirements in various populations" (36).

Table 8.14   Estimating Fluid Needs

mL/kg method
- 100 mL for first 10 kg of body weight
- 50 mL/kg for second 10 kg of body weight
- Age ≤ 50 years: 20 mL for each additional kg of body weight
- Age > 50 years: 15 mL for each additional kg of body weight

Body surface area method
- 1500 mL per square meter of body surface area

RDA method
- 1 mL fluid per kcal of estimated needs

Fluid balance method
- Urine output + 500 mL/d

Chronological age method
- Age 16–30 years (active): 40 mL/kg
- Age 20–55 years: 35 mL/kg
- Age 55–75 years: 30 mL/kg
- Age > 75 years: 25 mL/kg

Source: Data are from references 33 and 36.

VITAMIN AND MINERAL REQUIREMENTS: DIETARY REFERENCE INTAKES

According to the Institute of Medicine Food and Nutrition Board (37), "the Dietary Reference Intakes (DRIs) are a set of values that serve as standards for nutrient intakes for healthy persons in the United States and Canada." The following points from the Institute of Medicine are important to understanding the DRIs (37):

- The current values were established between 1997 and 2010. They cover 46 nutrient substances.
- DRI values are developed for different sex and age groups (and for pregnant and lactating women). Different groups have different DRI values.
- DRI values are based on average requirements (or average adverse intakes) and provide reliable information on the needs of groups of persons. However, because they are average values, DRIs cannot be used to ensure adequate or safe levels of intake for any single person. DRI values can be used as a guide for individuals but an individual's actual requirement or adverse intake level may be more or less than the DRI value.

The Institute of Medicine has categorized DRIs as follows (37):

- **Adequate Intake (AI)**: The recommended average daily intake level based on observed or experimentally determined approximations or estimates of nutrient intake by a group (or groups) of apparently healthy people that are assumed to be adequate; used when an RDA cannot be determined.
- **Estimated Average Requirement (EAR)**: The average daily nutrient intake level that is estimated to

meet the requirements of half the healthy individuals in a particular life stage and gender group.

- **Recommended Dietary Allowance (RDA)**: The average daily dietary nutrient intake level that is sufficient to meet the nutrient requirements of nearly all (97%–98%) healthy individuals in a particular life stage and gender group.
- **Tolerable Upper Intake Level (UL)**: The highest average daily nutrient intake level that is likely to pose no risk of adverse health effects to almost all individuals in the general population. As intake increases above the UL, the potential risk of adverse effects may increase.
- **Acceptable Macronutrient Distribution Ranges (AMDR)**: The range of intakes of an energy source that is associated with a reduced risk of chronic disease yet can provide adequate amounts of essential nutrients.

DRI tables published by the Institute of Medicine are available online (http://fnic.nal.usda.gov/dietary -guidance/dietary-reference-intakes/dri-tables-and -application-reports).

REFERENCES

1. Academy of Nutrition and Dietetics. eNCPT: Nutrition Care Process Terminology. 2014. https://ncpt.webauthor.com. Accessed April 13, 2015.
2. Academy of Nutrition and Dietetics Evidence Analysis Library. Adult Weight Management Evidence-Based Nutrition Practice Guideline. Determination of Resting Metabolic Rate. 2014. www.andeal.org/template.cfm?template=guide_summary &key=621. Accessed April 15, 2015.
3. Academy of Nutrition and Dietetics Evidence Analysis Library. Critical Illness (CI) Evidence-Based Nutrition Practice

Guideline. Determination of Resting Metabolic Rate (RMR). 2012. www.andeal.org/template.cfm?template=guide_summary &key=3200. Accessed April 15, 2015.

4. Mifflin MD, St. Jeor ST, Hill LA, Scott BJ, Daugherty SA, Koh YO. A new predictive equation for resting energy expenditure in healthy individuals. *Am J Clin Nutr.* 1990;51:241–247.

5. American Association for Respiratory Care (AARC). AARC clinical practice guideline. Metabolic measurement using indirect calorimetry during mechanical ventilation: 2004 revision and update. *Respir Care.* 2004;49(9):1073–1079.

6. Wooley JA, Sax, HC. Indirect calorimetry: Applications to practice. *Nutr Clin Pract.* 2003;18:434–439.

7. McClave SA, Lowen CC, Kleber MJ, McConnell ML, Jung LY, Goldsmith LJ. Clinical use of the respiratory quotient obtained from indirect calorimetry. *JPEN J Parenter Enteral Nutr.* 2003;27:21–26.

8. Academy of Nutrition and Dietetics Evidence Analysis Library. Critical Illness (CI) Evidence-Based Nutrition Practice Guideline. Respiratory Quotient as a Method to Detect Measurement Error. 2006. www.andeal.org/template.cfm?key=1006&cms _preview=1. Accessed April 15, 2015.

9. Wooley JA and Frankenfield D. Energy. In: Mueller C, ed. *The A.S.P.E.N. Adult Nutrition Support Core Curriculum.* 2nd ed. Silver Spring, MD: American Society for Parenteral and Enteral Nutrition; 2012:22–35.

10. Academy of Nutrition and Dietetics Evidence Analysis Library. Best Methods to Estimate RMR: Predictive Equation Formulas Used in Critically Ill Adults. 2010. www.andeal.org/topic .cfm?cat=4524. Accessed April 15, 2015.

11. Frankenfield DC, Coleman A, Alam S, Cooney RN. Analysis of estimation methods for resting metabolic rate in critically ill adults. *JPEN J Parenter Enteral Nutr.* 2009;33(1):27–35.

12. Frankenfield DC. Validation of an equation for resting metabolic rate in older obese critically ill patients. *JPEN J Parenter Enteral Nutr.* 2011;35:264–269.

13. Academy of Nutrition and Dietetics Evidence Analysis Library. Critical Illness. Hypocaloric, High Protein Feeding Regimen. 2012. www.andeal.org/template.cfm?template=guide _summary&key=3190. Accessed April 15, 2015.

14. Martindale RM, McClave SA, Vanek VW, et al. Guidelines for the provision and assessment of nutrition support therapy in the adult critically ill patient: Society of Critical Care Medicine and

American Society for Parenteral and Enteral Nutrition. *Crit Care Med.* 2009;37:1757–1761.

15. Choban PS, Burge JC, Scales D, Flancbaum L. Hypoenergetic nutrition support in hospitalized obese patients: A simplified method for clinical application. *Am J Clin Nutr.* 1997;66:546–550.

16. Frankenfield D, Ashcraft CM. Estimating energy needs in nutrition support patients. *JPEN J Parenter Enteral Nutr.* 2011;35:563–570.

17. Choban P, Dickerson R, Malone A, Worthington P, Compher C. A.S.P.E.N. Clinical guidelines: Nutrition support of hospitalized adult patients with obesity. *JPEN J Parenter Enteral Nutr.* 2013;37:714–744.

18. Dickerson RN. Hypocaloric feeding of obese patients in the intensive care unit. *Curr Opin Clin Nutr Metab Care.* 2005;8:189–196.

19. Shaw JH, Wildbore M, Wolf RR. Whole body protein kinetics in severely septic patients:The response to glucose infusion and total parenteral nutrition. *Ann Surg.* 1987;205:288–294.

20. Jacobs DG, Jacobs DO, Kudsk KA, Moore FA, Oswanski MF, Poole GV, Sacks G, Scherer LR 3rd, Sinclair KE. Practice management guidelines for nutrition support of trauma patients. *J Trauma.* 2004;57:660–679.

21. Young LS, Kearns LR, Schoefel SL, Clark NC. Protein. In: Mueller C, ed. *The A.S.P.E.N. Adult Nutrition Support Core Curriculum.* 2nd ed. Silver Spring, MD: American Society for Parenteral and Enteral Nutrition; 2012:83–97.

22. Choban PS, Dickerson RN. Morbid obesity and nutrition support: Is bigger different? *Nutr Clin Pract.* 2005;20:480–487.

23. Woulk R, Foulks C. Renal disease. In: Mueller C, ed. *The A.S.P.E.N. Adult Nutrition Support Core Curriculum.* 2nd ed. Silver Spring, MD: American Society for Parenteral and Enteral Nutrition; 2012:491–510.

24. Frazier TH, Wheeler BE, McClain CJ, Cave M. Liver Disease In: Mueller C, ed. *The A.S.P.E.N. Adult Nutrition Support Core Curriculum.* 2nd ed. Silver Spring, MD: American Society for Parenteral and Enteral Nutrition; 2012:454–471.

25. Mahan LK, Escott-Stump S. *Krause's Food, Nutrition, and Diet Therapy.* 12th ed. St. Louis, MO: WB Saunders; 2008.

26. Mahan K, Escott-Stump S, eds. *Krause's Food and the Nutrition Care Process.* 13th ed. Philadelphia, PA: WB Saunders; 2011.

27. Matarese L, Gottschlich M, eds. *Contemporary Nutrition Support Practice*. Philadelphia, PA: WB Saunders; 1998.

28. Gottschilch M, ed. *The A.S.P.E.N. Nutrition Support Core Curriculum: A Care-Based Approach—the Adult Patient*. Silver Spring, MD: American Society for Parenteral and Enteral Nutrition; 2007.

29. Plauth M, Cabre E, Riggio O, Assis-Camilo M, Pirlich M, Kondrup J, Ferenci P, Holm E, Vom Dahl S, Müller MJ, Nolte W. ESPEN guidelines on enteral nutrition: liver disease. *Clin. Nutr*. 2006;25:285–294.

30. Langley G, Tajchman S. Fluids, electrolytes, and acid-base disorders. In: Mueller C, ed. *The A.S.P.E.N. Adult Nutrition Support Core Curriculum*. 2nd ed. Silver Spring, MD: American Society for Parenteral and Enteral Nutrition; 2012:98–120.

31. Lucarelli MR, Pell LJ, Shirk MB, Mirtallo J. Fluid, electrolyte, and acid-base requirements. In: Cresci G, ed. *Nutrition Support for the Critically Ill Patient: A Guide to Practice*. Boca Raton FL: CRC Press; 2005:125–149.

32. Clary B, Milano C. *The Handbook of Surgical Intensive Care*. 5th ed. St. Louis, MO: Mosby; 2000.

33. Whitmire, SJ. Fluid, electrolytes, and acid-base balance. In: Matarese LE, Gottschlich MM. *Contemporary Nutrition Support Practice: A Clinical Guide*. 2nd ed. St. Louis, MO: WB Saunders; 2003:122–129.

34. Brown KA, Dickerson RN, Morgan LM, Alexander KH, Minard G, Brown RO. A new graduated dosing regimen for phosphorus replacement in patients receiving nutrition support. *JPEN J Parenter Enteral Nutr*. 2006;30:209–214.

35. Lyerly H, Gaynor J. *The Handbook of Surgical Intensive Care*. 3rd ed. St. Louis, MO: Mosby; 1992:410.

36. Academy of Nutrition and Dietetics Evidence Analysis Library. Hydration. Estimating Fluid Needs. www.andeal.org/topic.cfm?cat=3217&conclusion_statement_id=250894&highlight=fluid%20requirements&home=1. Accessed April 15, 2015.

37. Institute of Medicine. *Dietary Reference Intakes. The Essential Guide to Nutrient Requirements*. Washington, DC: National Academies Press; 2006. www.iom.edu/Reports/2006/Dietary-Reference-Intakes-Essential-Guide-Nutrient-Requirements.aspx. Accessed April 15, 2015.

Glossary

A1C: Glycated hemoglobin; used to assess the patient's mean plasma glucose level during the preceding two to three months

ABG: Arterial blood gas

acanthosis nigricans: Skin condition characterized by dark discoloration in body folds; associated with obesity and diabetes

ACD: *See* anemia of chronic disease (ACD)

ACE inhibitors: *See* angiotensin-converting enzyme (ACE) inhibitors

achlorhydria: Absence/deficiency of hydrochloric acid in gastric secretions

acid-base disorder: Change in the normal value of extracellular pH that may result when renal or respiratory function is abnormal or when an acid or base load overwhelms excretory capacity

acidosis: Excess acid in body fluids

acromegaly: Autonomous endocrine disease in which the pituitary gland produces excess growth hormone

activities of daily living (ADLs): Basic tasks of everyday life

acute respiratory distress syndrome: Syndrome caused by major lung injury, which leads to fluid in alveoli (air sacs) and prevents enough oxygen from getting to the lungs and into the blood

acute-phase response: Systemic response to acute or chronic inflammation associated with conditions such as infection, trauma, surgery, and cancer

Addison's disease: Adrenal insufficiency due to disorder of the adrenal glands

ADIME: Acronym for the steps of the Nutrition Care Process (Assessment, Diagnosis, Intervention, and Monitoring, and Evaluation)

adiposity: Obesity; fatness

ADL: *See* activities of daily living (ADLs)

AFA: *See* arm fat area (AFA)

AIDS: Acquired immunodeficiency syndrome

albumin: The major plasma protein

algorithm: Problem-solving method that uses answers to a series of yes/no questions to lead to diagnosis

alkalosis: Excess alkali (base) in body fluids

alopecia: Loss of hair; baldness

Alzheimer's disease: Irreversible brain disease that leads to memory loss and dementia

AMA: *See* arm muscle area (AMA)

amphetamines: Type of central nervous system-stimulant medications, which increase heart rate and blood pressure and decrease appetite

amyotrophic lateral sclerosis: Rapidly progressive, invariably fatal neurological disease that attacks the *neurons* responsible for controlling voluntary muscles

anabolism: The phase of metabolism in which simple substances are synthesized into the complex materials of living tissue

anasarca: Generalized massive edema

androgens: Male sex hormone compounds

anemia: Abnormally low number of red blood cells in the blood

anemia of chronic disease (ACD): Inability to use iron stores; typically mild and with a gradual onset after a malignant, infectious, inflammatory, or autoimmune condition. Therapy for ACD involves correcting the underlying disorder and use of erythropoietic agents.

angiotensin-converting enzyme (ACE) inhibitors: Group of medications that cause blood vessels to dilate, thereby reducing blood pressure

angular stomatitis: Sores or inflammation at the corners of the mouth

anion gap: The difference between the primary measured cation (sodium) and anions (chloride, bicarbonate). This difference or "gap" helps to determine the etiology of metabolic acidosis because it is increased when other unmeasured anions are present. Anion gap = (Sodium) − (Chloride + Bicarbonate)

anorexia nervosa: Eating disorder characterized by loss of weight greater than is considered healthy, distorted body image, and intense fear of gaining weight/becoming fat

anthropometry: The study of human body measurement, often for comparative purposes

antibiotics: Class of medicines that fight bacterial infections

anticonvulsants: Medications used to stop or control seizures

antihistamines: Class of medications that inhibit the action of histamine; used to treat allergies

antineoplastics: Class of drugs used to kill cancer cells

APACHE II: Tool used in intensive care to evaluate severity of disease

arm fat area (AFA): Indirect parameter of body composition calculated using triceps skinfold and arm circumference measurements; a person's AFA percentile may correspond to alterations in total body weight

arm muscle area (AMA): Indirect parameter of body composition calculated using triceps skinfold and arm circumference measurements; a person's AMA percentile may correspond to alterations in total body weight

arrhythmia: Irregular heartbeat

ascites: Accumulation of serous fluid in the abdominal cavity

Assessment, nutrition: First step in the Nutrition Care Process; an ongoing, nonlinear and dynamic process that involves data collection and continual analysis of the patient/client's nutritional status compared to specified criteria in order to identify nutrition-related problems, their causes, and significance

ataxia: Poor muscular coordination

atopic dermatitis: Chronic type of dermatitis; also called *allergic dermatitis*

atrophic lingual papillae: Slick tongue

auscultation: Listening for sounds within the body

azotemia: Disorder involving abnormally high levels of nitrogen-containing compounds (eg, urea, creatinine) in the blood, due in large part to renal dysfunction

barbiturates: Class of medications that depress the central nervous system; commonly used for their sedative effects

bariatric surgery: Procedure that alters the stomach and/or intestinal tract to help a person with obesity lose weight and reduce risk for obesity-related comorbidities

Bartter's syndrome: Type of congenital kidney defect that causes excessive urinary loss of sodium and calcium as well as potassium wasting

benzodiazepines: Class of medications used to treat anxiety and other psychological disorders

bezoar: Mass of swallowed foreign material (eg, hair) that is not digested and may cause blockage in the GI tract

BIA: *See* bioelectrical impedance analysis (BIA)

bile acid sequestrants: Lipid-lowering medications that work by binding to bile in the intestinal tract

bioelectrical impedance analysis (BIA): Tool that passes a small alternating current through the body to assess body composition

Bitot's spots: Superficial, triangular, foamy gray spots on the conjunctiva, consisting of keratinized epithelium

blood urea nitrogen (BUN): Amount of urea nitrogen in the blood; a BUN test evaluates renal function

BMI: *See* body mass index (BMI)

body mass index (BMI): Ratio of weight to height (kg/m^2) used as an estimate of body fat in the healthy population

bradycardia: Slower than normal heart rate; less than 60 pulses/min

bronchitis: Inflammation of the lining of the bronchial tubes; can be chronic or acute

bronchorrhea: Excessive discharge of mucus from the bronchi

bulimia nervosa: Type of eating disorder characterized by repeated episodes of bingeing and purging

cachexia: Profound state of muscle and fat wasting

Calorie count: *See* Nutrient intake record (calorie count)

CAM: *See* complementary and alternative medicine (CAM)

cathartics: Medications that cause the emptying of the bowels/defecation

CBW: Current body weight

ceruloplasmin: Copper-containing protein in the blood

cheilosis: Dry, cracking, ulcerated lips

cholinergics: Drugs that produce the same effect as the neurohormone acetylcholine

Chvostek's sign: Twitch of the facial muscles upon tapping the facial nerve in front of the ear; twitching is due to neuromuscular excitability secondary to hypocalcemia

cirrhosis: Disease caused by the slow accumulation of scar tissue in the liver, which prevents normal hepatic functions

CMS: Centers for Medicare & Medicaid Services

cobalamin: Vitamin B-12

colonic interposition: Esophagectomy (surgical procedure to replace the esophagus) in which part of the colon is used as the replacement

complementary and alternative medicine (CAM): Medical practices and products that are not part of standard care provided by physicians and allied health care providers; complementary medicine is provided along with standard care; alternative medicine is provided instead of standard care

computerized tomography (CT): Imaging technique that uses X-ray to produce images of the different tissues in the body; used to estimate whole and regional body composition

congenital adrenal hyperplasia: Any of a group of autosomal recessive disorders that involve a deficiency of an enzyme that helps synthesize cortisol, aldosterone, or both

conjunctiva: Membrane that lines the eyelids and covers the exposed surface of the sclera

COPD: Chronic obstructive pulmonary disease

corticosteroids: Class of medications that closely resemble the adrenal hormone cortisol; used to suppress inflammation (eg, in asthma)

costochondral beading/rachitic rosary: Prominent, beadlike knobs on bones in the rib cage; a sign of rickets

crackles: Discontinuous breath sounds. Fine crackles are "popping" noises. Coarse crackles are lower pitched and more noticeable on expiration

C-reactive protein: Type of plasma protein; the most predominant of the acute-phase proteins

creatinine: Byproduct of creatine phosphate breakdown in muscle; blood or urine tests of creatinine levels can help assess renal function

CT: *See* computerized tomography (CT)

Cushing's syndrome: Autonomous endocrine disease involving exposure to high levels of cortisol

cystic fibrosis: Genetic disorder that affects the lungs as well as the pancreas and liver

cytokines: Types of proteins that are released by a cell population on contact with a specific antigen, to act as intercellular mediators (eg, in an immune response)

decubitus: The position of lying down

decubitus ulcers: Pressure ulcers / "bed sores."

dehydration: The clinical consequences of losing excess free water; not to be confused with *hypovolemia* (a loss of water and sodium leading to extracellular fluid [ECF] volume contraction)

delayed cutaneous hypersensitivity: Skin test formerly used to quantify the impaired immune function associated with uncomplicated malnutrition

dementia: General loss of cognitive abilities, including the impairment of memory, severe enough to impair activities of daily living

dermatitis: Inflammation of the skin

desquamation: Exfoliation; shedding of skin

DETERMINE Checklist: Nutritional risk screening tool for elderly adults. DETERMINE stands for Disease, Eating poorly, Tooth loss/mouth pain, Economic hardship, Reduced social contact, Multiple medications, Involuntary weight loss/gain, Needs assistance in self-care, Elder years > age 80

diabetes insipidus: Uncommon condition in which the kidneys are unable to prevent the excretion of water

diabetes mellitus: State of chronic hyperglycemia resulting from a deficiency of insulin and/or resistance to the action of insulin

diabetic ketoacidosis: Serious complication of diabetes characterized by high levels of ketones in the blood

Diagnosis, nutrition: Second step in the Nutrition Care Process; the nutrition diagnosis identifies and describes a specific nutrition problem that can be resolved or improved through treatment/nutrition intervention by a dietetics practitioner. A nutrition diagnosis (eg, inconsistent carbohydrate intake) is different from a medical diagnosis (eg, diabetes)

diarrhea: Having frequent, loose watery stools (>3 times/d)

diastolic blood pressure: The bottom number in the blood pressure measurement; measures the pressure in the arteries between heart beats

diurnal variation: Fluctuation during a day

dual energy X-ray absorptiometry (DXA): Noninvasive method of direct measurement of the three components of body composition (water, protein, and fat)

dumping syndrome: Reaction secondary to excessively rapid emptying of gastric contents into the jejunum, which occurs after ingestion of food in patients who have had part or all of their stomach removed; symptoms can include cramps, nausea, weakness, sweating, palpitation, and diarrhea

DXA: *See* dual energy X-ray absorptiometry (DXA)

dyspnea: Breathlessness or shortness of breath

ecchymosis: Small hemorrhagic spot, which is a nonelevated, rounded, or irregular blue or purplish patch in the skin or mucous membranes; larger than a petechia

ECF: *See* extracellular fluid volume (ECF)

edema: Much larger than normal amounts of fluids in the intracellular tissue spaces of the body

EHR: Electronic health record

EKG: Electrocardiogram

emesis: The process of vomiting

emphysema: Type of chronic obstructive pulmonary disease that damages the alveoli (air sacs)

EN: *See* enteral nutrition (EN)

enteral nutrition (EN): Delivery of nutrition through a feeding tube into the stomach or small intestine

enterocutaneous fistula: Abnormal connection between the large or small bowel and the skin

erythrocyte sedimentation rate (ESR): Blood test used to indirectly measure inflammation in the body

ESR: *See* erythrocyte sedimentation rate (ESR)

exhaustive thinking: Gathering of as much data as possible followed by search through data for any and all possible diagnoses

extracellular fluid volume (ECF): A measurement of the body's volume status

Fanconi syndrome: Disorder of the kidney tubes in which certain substances normally absorbed into the bloodstream by the kidneys are released into the urine instead; may or may not be congenital

fat-free mass (FFM): Total body mass minus the fat; used to assess body composition

ferritin: Intracellular protein that stores iron

FFM: *See* fat-free mass (FFM)

fistula: Abnormal connection between an organ, vessel, or intestine and another structure

flag sign: Transverse pigmentation of hair

flail chest: Injury in which a segment of the thoracic cage is separated from the rest of the chest wall, preventing the injured part from contributing to lung expansion; indicates an underlying pulmonary contusion

follicular hyperkeratosis: Skin condition characterized by excessive development of keratin in hair follicles; looks like "goose bumps" but the bumps do not go away with warming or rubbing

food diary: Record of food and nutrient intake for a set period of time, kept by the patient/client or caregiver

food frequency questionnaire: Questionnaire for determining food and nutrient intake

gastrectomy: Removal of part or all of the stomach

gastric banding: Type of bariatric procedure in which a band is used to restrict the capacity of the stomach

gastric pull-up: Esophagectomy (surgical procedure to replace the esophagus) in which part of the stomach is used as the replacement

gastroesophageal reflux disease (GERD): Condition in which the stomach contents (food or liquid) leak backwards from the stomach into the esophagus

gastroparesis: Muscular dysfunction in the stomach that delays or prevents digestion

gender: The Institute of Medicine defines gender as "a person's self-representation as male or female, or how that person is responded to by social institutions based on the individual's gender presentation." *See also* sex

GERD: *See* gastroesophageal reflux disease (GERD)

glomerulonephritis: Type of kidney disease in which the glomeruli are damaged, causing blood and protein to be lost in urine

glucagonoma: Rare neuroendocrine tumor of the pancreas

glucosuria: Glucose excreted in urine

Guillain-Barré syndrome: Neuromuscular disorder in which the body's immune system attacks part of the peripheral nervous system. Symptoms range from mild tingling in extremities to total paralysis

Hamwi formula: Equation (not validated) used to estimate ideal body weight in a clinical setting

heart murmur: Swishing or blowing sound resulting from altered blood flow in the heart

hematocrit: Blood test to measure the percentage of whole blood volume made up of red blood cells

hemochromatosis: Type of iron-overload disease

hemoconcentration: Increased concentration of cells and solids in the blood, often due to hypovolemia

hemolysis: Breakdown of red blood cells

hemolytic anemia: Anemia caused by the bone marrow failing to replace red blood cells that are being destroyed

hemothorax: Collection of blood in the pleural cavity (space between chest wall and lung)

hepatomegaly: Enlargement of the liver

HHS: *See* hyperosmolar hyperglycemic state (HHS)

HIV: Human immunodeficiency virus

HMG CoA reductase inhibitors: Statin drugs; used to lower serum cholesterol levels

homeostatic mechanisms: Mechanisms activated by negative feedback that contribute to the tendency of an organism or cell to regulate its internal conditions (homeostasis)

hungry bone syndrome: Disorder that occurs in some patients after a parathyroidectomy and is characterized by rapid/excessive osteogenesis that can result in hypocalcemia

hyperaldosteronism: Excess of the hormone aldosterone, which is secreted by the adrenal gland

hypercalcemia: Abnormally high serum calcium level

hypercapnia: High concentration of carbon dioxide in the blood (PCO_2 >45 mmHg)

hyperchloremia: Abnormally high serum chloride level

hyperchloremic acidosis: Type of metabolic acidosis that occurs when there is an excessive loss of sodium bicarbonate from the body (eg, with severe diarrhea)

hyperglycemia: Abnormally high blood glucose level (>140 mg/dL in hospital setting)

hyperkalemia: Abnormally high serum potassium level

hyperlipidemia: Abnormally high blood lipid levels

hypermagnesemia: Abnormally high serum magnesium level

hypernatremia: Abnormally high serum sodium level (>145 mEq/L)

hyperosmolar hyperglycemic state (HHS): Serious complication of diabetes characterized by hyperglycemia, hyperosmolarity, and dehydration without significant ketoacidosis

hyperosmolar hyponatremia: Hyponatremia with elevated serum osmolality

hyperparathyroidism: Disorder involving secretion of abnormally high levels of parathyroid hormone (PTH)

hyperphosphatemia: Abnormally high serum phosphate levels

hypertension: Blood pressure >140 mmHg/90 mmHg

hyperthermia: Abnormally high body temperature

hyperthyroidism: Overactive thyroid gland

hypervolemia: A state of extracellular fluid (ECF) volume expansion

hypervolemic hypernatremia: Total-body sodium excess greater than total-body water excess (uncommon)

hypervolemic hypotonic hyponatremia: Excess total-body sodium with larger excess of total-body water

hypoalbuminemia: Abnormally low serum albumin levels

hypocalcemia: Abnormally low serum calcium level

hypodypsia: Abnormally reduced sense of thirst

hypogeusia: Decreased sense of taste

hypoglycemia: Abnormally low blood glucose level (eg, <70 mg/dL)

hypokalemia: Abnormally low serum potassium level

hypomagnesemia: Abnormally low serum magnesium level

hyponatremia: Abnormally low serum sodium level (<135 mEq/L)

hypoparathyroidism: Disorder involving secretion of abnormally low levels of parathyroid hormone (PTH)

hypoperfusion: Decreased blood flow through an organ

hyporeflexia: Reduced functioning of the reflexes

hyposmia: Decreased sense of smell

hypotension: Abnormally low blood pressure

hypothermia: Abnormally low body temperature

hypothetico-deductive reasoning: Problem-solving method in which a list of possible diagnoses is developed and altered as information gathering progresses

hypothyroidism: Insufficient level/production of thyroid hormone

hypovolemia: Decrease in the volume of circulating blood

hypovolemia: Loss of water and sodium leading to extracellular fluid (ECF) volume contraction; not to be confused with *dehydration* (the clinical consequences of losing excess free water)

hypovolemic hypernatremia: Total-body sodium deficit with larger total-body water deficit

hypovolemic hypotonic hyponatremia: Total-body water deficit with larger total-body sodium deficit

hypoxemia: Abnormally low blood oxygen

hypoxia: Failure of oxygenation at the tissue level

iatrogenic: Inadvertently resulting from medical treatment, therapy, or procedure

IBD: *See* inflammatory bowel disease (IBD)

IBS: *See* irritable bowel syndrome (IBS)

IBW: *See* ideal body weight (IBW)

IDA: *See* iron-deficiency anemia (IDA)

ideal body weight (IBW): Historically, the weight associated with the lowest mortality determined by actuarial data from life insurance companies; also sometimes defined as a weight that would fall within the "normal" range for body mass index or as a weight estimated using an IBW formula based on height, sex, and possibly frame size

IDNT: *See* International Dietetics and Nutrition Terminology (IDNT)

ileocecal valve: Valve between the small and large intestines that keeps material from flowing back into the small intestine after it enters the large

ileus: A disruption of the normal propulsive ability of the gastrointestinal tract

inflammatory bowel disease (IBD): Chronic inflammation of all or part of the gastrointestinal tract; types of IBD include ulcerative colitis and Crohn's disease

inspection: The gathering of data via close observation

insulinoma: Pancreatic tumor that secretes insulin

International Dietetics and Nutrition Terminology (IDNT): Former name for the standardized terminology now called Nutrition Care Process Terminology (NCPT)

interstitial fluid: Fluid in spaces between cells in tissues

Intervention, nutrition: The third step in the Nutrition Care Process; a purposefully planned action intended to positively change a nutrition-related behavior, environmental condition, or aspect of health status for an individual (and his/her family or caregivers), target group, or the community at large

intrinsic factor: Protein used by the intestine to absorb vitamin B-12

iron-deficiency anemia (IDA): Anemia caused when body has insufficient iron to create normal levels of red blood cells

irritable bowel syndrome (IBS): Common disorder of the colon characterized by cramping, gas, constipation, and/or diarrhea, but not involving inflammation

iso-osmolar hyponatremia: Hyponatremia with normal serum osmolality

isovolemic hypernatremia: Total-body water loss with normal total-body sodium

isovolemic hypotonic hyponatremia: Normal to moderately increased total-body water ± total-body sodium

jaundice: Yellow (bile pigment) discoloration of skin, mucous membranes, and sclera as a result of elevated serum bilirubin

ketoacidosis: Type of metabolic acidosis characterized by a high concentration of ketones. *See also* diabetic ketoacidosis

koilonychia: Dystrophy of the fingernails resulting in thin, concave nails with the edges raised. Also called "spoon nail"; associated with iron deficiency

Korsakoff's psychosis: Permanent damage to areas of the brain involved with memory caused by thiamin deficiency

kwashiorkor: A severe type of protein-energy malnutrition most often affecting young children, particularly in areas of famine; rare in developed nations

kyphoscoliosis: A type of spinal deformity involving outward and lateral curvature

lactic acidosis: Persistently high levels of lactic acid in association with metabolic acidosis

leukemia: Cancer of the bone marrow that affects white blood cell production

leukocytosis: Disorder characterized by excessive number of white blood cells

loop diuretics: Diuretic medications that work in the loop of Henle; may be used to treat heart failure, hypertension, and edema

lymphoma: Cancer of the lymph system

MAC: *See* midarm circumference (MAC)

Malnutrition Screening Tool (MST): Rapid nutritional risk screen that can be completed, by nurses or other ancillary personnel, when a patient is admitted to acute or ambulatory care

Malnutrition Universal Screening Tool (MUST): Nutritional risk screening tool that uses an assessment of the severity of illness and body mass index

MAMC: *See* arm muscle area (AMA)

MAOI: *See* monoamine oxidase inhibitors (MAOIs)

marasmus: Severe type of protein-energy malnutrition seen in children who experience prolonged, severe energy deficit in the first year of life; rare in developed nations

MCT: Medium-chain triglyceride

MCV: *See* mean corpuscular volume (MCV)

MDS: *See* Minimum Data Set (MDS)

Meals on Wheels: Network of volunteer programs that home-deliver meals to senior citizens

mean corpuscular volume (MCV): Measurement of the average size of red blood cells

megaloblastic anemias: Vitamin B-12- or folate-deficiency anemia

metabolic acid-base disorder: Acid-base disorder that manifests as changes in serum chloride and bicarbonate (HCO_3). The body attempts to compensate for a primary metabolic acid-base disorder with "secondary" or "compensatory" respiratory changes

metabolic acidosis: Acidosis that occurs when the kidneys cannot eliminate acid buildup or when the body excretes too much base

metabolic alkalosis: Alkalosis caused by too much bicarbonate in the blood; may be associated with renal disease

methylmalonic acid (MMA): Substance produced when amino acids in the body break down; serum MMA is measured to assess vitamin B-12-deficiency anemia

midarm circumference (MAC): Measurement of the circumference of the upper arm at the midpoint between the acromion process of the scapula and the olecranon process of the ulna; used in the assessment of body composition/muscle protein

midarm muscle circumference (MAMC): *See* arm muscle area (AMA)

Minimum Data Set (MDS): Primary screening and assessment tool published by the Centers for Medicare & Medicaid Services (CMS) for use in long-term care facilities. The MDS contains items that measure physical, psychological, and psychosocial functioning.

Mini Nutritional Assessment (MNA): Nutritional risk screening tool published by Nestlé for use with elderly patients/clients in long-term care settings; formerly known as Mini Nutritional Assessment Short Form (MNA-SF)

MNA: *See* Mini Nutritional Assessment (MNA)

Monitoring and evaluation, nutrition: The fourth step of the Nutrition Care Process; nutrition monitoring and evaluation aims to determine and measure the amount of progress made for the nutrition intervention and whether the nutrition-related goals or expected outcomes are being met. Monitoring and evaluation help promote more uniformity within the dietetics profession in assessing the effectiveness of nutrition intervention.

monoamine oxidase inhibitors (MAOIs): Class of antidepressant medications

MST: *See* Malnutrition Screening Tool (MST)

multiple myeloma: Cancer of plasma cells

multiple sclerosis: Abnormal immune-mediated response directed against myelin and nerve fibers in the central nervous system, which causes interruptions in the communication between the spinal cord, nerves, and brain

muscular dystrophy: Group of more than 30 genetic diseases characterized by progressive weakness and degeneration of the skeletal muscles that control movement

MUST: *See* Malnutrition Universal Screening Tool (MUST)

myalgia: Muscle pain

myasthenia gravis: Chronic autoimmune neuromuscular disease characterized by varying degrees of weakness of the skeletal (voluntary) muscles of the body, with weakness increasing after activity and decreasing with rest

NCP: *See* Nutrition Care Process (NCP)

NCPM: *See* Nutrition Care Process Model (NCPM)

NCPT: *See* Nutrition Care Process Terminology (NCPT)

necrosis: Death of body tissue

neoplasm: Tumor; abnormal mass of tissue that results when cells divide more than they should or do not die when they should

NPO: *Nil per os* (nothing by mouth); instruction to withhold oral intake of food and fluids

NRS-2002: *See* Nutrition Risk Score (NRS-2002)

NSAID: Nonsteroidal anti-inflammatory drug

Nutrient intake record (calorie count): Recording of actual nutrient consumption via direct observation or tray audit

Nutrition Care Process (NCP): Process for identifying, planning for, and meeting nutritional needs. Includes four steps: nutrition assessment, nutrition diagnosis, nutrition intervention, nutrition monitoring and evaluation

Nutrition Care Process Model (NCPM): Graphic visualization that illustrates the steps of the Nutrition Care Process (NCP) and the internal and external factors that impact use of the NCP. The screening and referral and outcomes management systems referenced in the

NCPM are outside the nutrition care steps managed
directly by the RDN.

Nutrition Care Process Terminology (NCPT): Standardized language used to describe, document, and record nutrition and dietetics practice

Nutrition Risk Score (NRS-2002): Tool used to evaluate whether patients need enteral or parenteral nutrition support

oliguria: Reduced urine output in relation to fluid intake

ophthalmoplegia: Paralysis of the ocular muscles

opiates: Class of medications used to treat pain

orthostatic hypotension: Rapid drop in blood pressure of 25 mmHg when changing from supine to sitting or standing position (associated with hypovolemia)

osmolality: Particles per kilogram of water

osmolarity: Particles per liter of solution

osteomalcia: Softening of the bones caused by vitamin D deficiency

osteoporosis: Decrease in amount of bone mass that increases risks of fractures and other bone problems

ostomy: Surgery to create an opening (stoma) from an area inside the body to the outside

palpation: Using the hands, fingertips, and finger pads to apply light to deep pressure to the skin to determine structures beneath the surface and to detect abnormalities

pancreatectomy: Surgical removal of all or part of the pancreas

pancreatic insufficiency: Deficiency of exocrine pancreatic enzymes that results in maldigestion

pancreaticoduodenectomy: Surgical procedure to remove malignancies from the pancreas, duodenum, and related organs

pancreatitis: Inflammation of the pancreas

paracentesis: Procedure to aspirate fluid from the abdomen or other body cavity; may be used for diagnostic or therapeutic purposes

paralytic ileus: Paralysis of the intestine

paraplegia: Paralysis of the lower half of the body

parenteral nutrition (PN): Nutrition given into the blood through an intravenous tube into a vein

paresthesias: Sudden numbness, burning, pricking (pins and needles), or itching sensation in the skin

parotid enlargement: Swelling of the major salivary gland

pattern recognition: Decision making based on past experience with similar cases

PCO_2: Partial pressure of carbon dioxide in the blood

PCOS: *See* polycystic ovary syndrome (PCOS)

percussion: The act of striking one object against another to produce vibration and sound waves; percussion data from the medical record may be relevant to nutrition assessment

pericardial friction rub: Squeaky or rubbing heart sound, caused by inflamed layers of the pericardium rubbing against each other

peristalsis: Series of muscle contractions in the gastrointestinal tract that move food through the digestive system

peritonitis: Bacterial or fungal infection of the peritoneum, a tissue that lines the inner abdomen and covers the abdominal organs

PES statement: Method for structuring a nutrition diagnosis. PES is an abbreviation for "problem, etiology, signs and symptoms," and the PES statement is written in the form "Problem [the specific diagnosis] *related to* etiology [the specific cause(s)] *as evidenced*

by signs and symptoms [the key abnormal findings that determined the diagnosis]."

petechia: Pinpoint, nonelevated, round, purplish-red spot, which occurs with intradermal or submucosal hemorrhage

pH: A measure of acidity/alkalinity based on the number of hydrogen ions (H+) present

phenothiazines: Class of tranquilizing/antipsychotic medications

pheochromocytoma: Rare tumor of the adrenal gland

Pickwickian syndrome: Obesity hypoventilation syndrome; a disorder in people with obesity in which poor breathing leads to lower oxygen and higher carbon dioxide levels in the blood

"pigeon" chest: Horizontal depression along the lower border of chest

pleural friction rub: Lung sounds that vary from a few intermittent sounds similar to crackles to harsh grating, creaking, or leathery sounds that occur with respiration

PMH: Past medical history

PN: *See* parenteral nutrition (PN)

pneumothorax: Total collapse of the lung

polycystic ovary syndrome (PCOS): Hormonal disorder that affects women of reproductive age, causing menstrual irregularities and problems with fertility/ conception

polycythemia vera: Rare bone marrow disorder that leads to overproduction of blood cells, especially red blood cells

polydipsia: Excessive thirst

polyphagia: Excessive hunger/increased appetite

polyuria: Excessive urination

prealbumin: Transport protein for thyroxin (thyroid hormone). Also, when combined with retinol-binding protein, transports vitamin A. Also known as "transthyretin"

prescription, nutrition: The patient's or client's individual recommended dietary intake of energy and/or selected foods or nutrients based on current reference standards and dietary guidelines and the patient's or client's specified health and nutrition diagnosis

prokinetic agents: Class of drugs that increases gastrointestinal motility; used in various gastrointestinal disorders

proteinuria: Abnormally high amount of protein in urine, a sign of chronic kidney disease

pseudohyponatremia: Artifactually low serum sodium concentration related to certain laboratory techniques; does not warrant treatment

pulmonary artery occlusion pressure: Procedure used to evaluate pulmonary edema; a measurement of pressure in a small pulmonary arterial branch

purpura: Any of a group of conditions characterized by ecchymoses or other small hemorrhages in the skin or mucous membranes

QOL: *See* quality of life (QOL)

quadriplegia: Paralysis of the entire body below the neck or of all four limbs

quality of life (QOL): Patient/client-centered measure of the patient's/client's social, physical, emotional, and mental well-being. Nutrition may affect quality of life.

rachitic rosary: *See* costochondral beading/rachitic rosary

RDW: *See* red cell distribution width (RDW)

red blood cell folate: Test to assess megaloblastic anemia

red cell distribution width (RDW): Measurement of variation in red blood cell size or red blood cell volume

refeeding syndrome: Potentially fatal metabolic shifts in fluids and electrolytes that may occur in malnourished patients receiving nutrition support (enteral or parenteral)

renal dysplasia: Congenital disorder of the kidney in which normal kidney tissue is replaced by cysts

renal tubular acidosis: Disorder in which the kidneys fail to sufficiently excrete acids in the urine, leading to excessive levels of acid in the blood

reset osmostat syndrome: Disorder in which kidneys can concentrate and dilute urine appropriately but the threshold for antidiuretic hormone (ADH) secretion is reset to a lower-than-normal value, thus resulting in hyponatremia

respiratory acid-base disorder: Acid-base disorder that is characterized by abnormalities in partial pressure of carbon dioxide in the blood (PCO_2). Primary respiratory acid-base disorder typically elicits a compensatory renal response.

respiratory acidosis: Acidosis that develops when there is too much carbon dioxide in the body; usually caused when the body is unable to remove enough carbon dioxide through breathing

respiratory alkalosis: Alkalosis caused by low levels of carbon dioxide in the blood

retinol-binding protein: Type of plasma protein that transports retinol to the peripheral tissues

rhabdomyolysis: Breakdown of muscle tissue that leads to the release of myoglobin into the blood; can cause renal damage

rhoncus: Snoring sound caused by secretions in the trachea or bronchi

rickets: Disorder caused by a lack of vitamin D, calcium, or phosphate, which leads to softening and weakening of the bones

RLQ: Right lower quadrant, the location of the ileocecal valve

Roux-en-Y gastric bypass: Type of bariatric procedure in which a stomach pouch is created out of a small portion of the stomach and attached directly to the small intestine, bypassing a large part of the stomach and duodenum. The pouch restricts the volume of food intake, and bypass of the duodenum reduces fat absorption.

sacral edema: Edema in the region of the sacrum, the triangular bone just below the lumbar vertebrae

salt-wasting nephropathy: Intrinsic renal disease causing abnormal urinary sodium loss

scaphoid abdomen: Abdomen that appears sunken/concave

sclera: White of the eye

screening, nutrition: Process of identifying patients, clients, or groups who may have a nutrition diagnosis and benefit from nutrition assessment and intervention by a registered dietitian nutritionist (RDN). Patients/clients enter nutrition assessment, the first step of the Nutrition Care Process (NCP), through screening, surveillance systems data, and/or referral, all of which are outside of the NCP

seborrhea: Scaling of skin around nostrils

sepsis: Severe infection in which release of immunological agents leads to inflammation throughout the body

sex: The Institute of Medicine defines sex as "the classification of living things, generally as male or female, according to their reproductive organs and functions assigned by chromosomal complement." *See also* gender

SIADH: *See* syndrome of inappropriate antidiuretic hormone (SIADH)

sickle cell anemia: Genetic disease in which the body produces crescent-/sickle-shaped red blood cells; symptoms include anemia and pain

sleep apnea: Chronic disorder in which shallow breathing or pauses in breathing interrupts sleep

sleeve gastrectomy: Type of bariatric procedure in which a large portion of the stomach is removed

SNAQ: Short Nutritional Assessment Questionnaire

soluble transferrin receptor (sTfR): Laboratory value that is useful to distinguish between iron-deficiency anemia and anemia of chronic disease

sorbitol: Type of sugar alcohol; used as an artificial sweetener

Special Supplemental Nutrition Program for Women, Infants, and Children (WIC): State-run program using federal grants to provide supplemental foods, health care referrals, and nutrition education for low-income pregnant, breastfeeding, and non-breastfeeding postpartum women, and to infants and children up to age five who are found to be at nutritional risk

spider angioma: Abnormal collection of blood vessels near the skin; the lesion has reddish extensions that move out from a center point

stadiometer/statiometer: Measuring rod used to assess height

steatorrhea: Presence of fat in stools as a result of fat malabsorption

sTfR: *See* soluble transferrin receptor (sTfR)

sulfonylureas: Class of drugs used to increase insulin release from the pancreas and manage type 2 diabetes

syndrome of inappropriate antidiuretic hormone (SIADH): Syndrome of inappropriate antidiuretic hormone (ADH) secretion, characterized by hypertonic urine output, normal glomerular filtration rate, normal or expanded (no edema) total body water, urinary sodium wasting, hypoosmolality, hyponatremia, and increased antidiuretic hormone (ADH) release

systolic blood pressure: Top number in the blood pressure measurement; measures the pressure in the arteries when the heart beats

tachycardia: Faster than normal heart rate; more than 100 pulses/min

TCAs: *See* tricyclic antidepressants (TCAs)

tendon reflex: Stretch reflex caused by a blow to a muscle tendon; test is used to assess spinal cord and neuromuscular integrity

tetany: Hyperexcitability of nerves and muscles due to decrease in concentration of extracellular ionized calcium; characterized by muscular twitching or cramping

thiazides: Class of diuretic medications

thrombocytopenia: Decrease in the number of platelets

thrombocytopenia: Disorder in which platelet levels are abnormally low

thrombocytosis: Disorder characterized by excessive number of platelets in the blood

TIBC: *See* total iron-binding capacity (TIBC)

total iron-binding capacity (TIBC): Blood test used to measure iron in blood

total lymphocyte count: Test formerly used to quantify the impaired immune function associated with uncomplicated malnutrition

transferrin: Plasma protein that binds and transports iron

transferrin saturation (TSAT): Blood test to measure the percentage of serum iron that is bound to transferrin (ie, the amount of iron available to tissues)

transthyretin: *See* prealbumin

triceps skinfold (TSF): Indirect index of body fat stores; TSF is measured using skinfold calipers on the midline posterior surface of the arm over the triceps muscle, at the midpoint between the acromion process of the scapula and the olecranon process of the ulna

tricyclic antidepressants (TCAs): Class of medications used to treat depression

Trousseau's sign: Hand spasm observed when the blood pressure cuff is inflated to above systolic blood pressure for up to three minutes; the muscular contractions are due to neuromuscular excitability secondary to hypocalcemia

TSAT: *See* transferrin saturation (TSAT)

TSF: *See* triceps skinfold (TSF)

tumor lysis syndrome: Group of metabolic complications (hyperuricemia, hyperkalemia, hyperphosphatemia, hypocalcemia, and acute renal failure) that can follow anticancer treatment

24-hour recall: Interview method for determining food and nutrient intake

tympany: Drum- or bell-like sound created when percussion is performed over an air-filled cavity

UBW: *See* usual body weight (UBW)

ulcerative colitis: Type of inflammatory bowel disease affecting the colon and rectum

ureterosigmoidostomy: Surgical diversion of ureters to the sigmoid colon

urine specific gravity: Laboratory test of the concentration of chemical particles in urine; used to assess hydration status

usual body weight (UBW): An individual's typical weight, based on weight history; used in assessment of weight change

vagotomy: Resection of the vagus nerve (the nerve that causes acid secretion to the stomach)

vasodilation: Widening of the blood vessels

villous adenoma: Type of polyp (sometimes malignant) in the colon or other parts of the gastrointestinal tract

weight pattern: Changes in weight (often measured as percentages) over time

Wernicke-Korsakoff syndrome: Brain disorder due to thiamin deficiency

Whipple procedure: *See* pancreaticoduodenectomy

WIC: *See* Special Supplemental Nutrition Program for Women, Infants, and Children (WIC)

xerosis: Abnormal dryness of the eye

Index

Page number followed by *t* indicates table, by *f* indicates figure.